Marine Sediments

Marine Sediments

Processes, Transport and Environmental Aspects

Special Issue Editors

Marcello Di Risio
Donald F. Hayes
Davide Pasquali

MDPI • Basel • Beijing • Wuhan • Barcelona • Belgrade

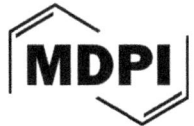

Special Issue Editors

Marcello Di Risio
University of L'Aquila
Italy

Donald F. Hayes
University of Nevada
USA

Davide Pasquali
University of L'Aquila
Italy

Editorial Office
MDPI
St. Alban-Anlage 66
4052 Basel, Switzerland

This is a reprint of articles from the Special Issue published online in the open access journal *Journal of Marine Science and Engineering* (ISSN 2077-1312) from 2019 to 2020 (available at: https://www.mdpi.com/journal/jmse/special_issues/mar.sediment).

For citation purposes, cite each article independently as indicated on the article page online and as indicated below:

LastName, A.A.; LastName, B.B.; LastName, C.C. Article Title. *Journal Name* **Year**, *Article Number*, Page Range.

ISBN 978-3-03943-396-4 (Hbk)
ISBN 978-3-03943-397-1 (PDF)

Cover image courtesy of Marcello Di Risio.

© 2020 by the authors. Articles in this book are Open Access and distributed under the Creative Commons Attribution (CC BY) license, which allows users to download, copy and build upon published articles, as long as the author and publisher are properly credited, which ensures maximum dissemination and a wider impact of our publications.

The book as a whole is distributed by MDPI under the terms and conditions of the Creative Commons license CC BY-NC-ND.

Contents

About the Special Issue Editors vii

Marcello Di Risio, Donald F. Hayes and Davide Pasquali
Marine Sediments: Processes, Transport and Environmental Aspects
Reprinted from: *J. Mar. Sci. Eng.* **2020**, *8*, 243, doi:10.3390/jmse8040243 1

Dechao Hu, Min Wang, Shiming Yao and Zhongwu Jin
Study on the Spillover of Sediment during Typical Tidal Processes in the Yangtze Estuary Using a High-Resolution Numerical Model
Reprinted from: *J. Mar. Sci. Eng.* **2019**, *7*, 390, doi:10.3390/jmse7110390 4

Fotini Botsou, Aristomenis P. Karageorgis, Vasiliki Paraskevopoulou, Manos Dassenakis and Michael Scoullos
Critical Processes of Trace Metals Mobility in Transitional Waters: Implications from the Remote, Antinioti Lagoon, Corfu Island, Greece
Reprinted from: *J. Mar. Sci. Eng.* **2019**, *7*, 307, doi:10.3390/jmse7090307 28

Markes E. Johnson, Rigoberto Guardado-France, Erlend M. Johnson and Jorge Ledesma-Vázquez
Geomorphology of a Holocene Hurricane Deposit Eroded from Rhyolite Sea Cliffs on Ensenada Almeja (Baja California Sur, Mexico)
Reprinted from: *J. Mar. Sci. Eng.* **2019**, *7*, 193, doi:10.3390/jmse7060193 53

Iolanda Lisi, Alessandra Feola, Antonello Bruschi, Andrea Pedroncini, Davide Pasquali and Marcello Di Risio
Mathematical Modeling Framework of Physical Effects Induced by Sediments Handling Operations in Marine and Coastal Areas
Reprinted from: *J. Mar. Sci. Eng.* **2019**, *7*, 149, doi:10.3390/jmse7050149 75

Olga Kuznetsova and Yana Saprykina
Influence of Underwater Bar Location on Cross-Shore Sediment Transport in the Coastal Zone
Reprinted from: *J. Mar. Sci. Eng.* **2019**, *7*, 55, doi:10.3390/jmse7030055 101

About the Special Issue Editors

Marcello Di Risio is the associate professor of Maritime and Hydraulic Structures at the Department of Civil, Construction-Architectural and Environmental Engineering of the University of L'Aquila (Italy). He is the head of the Environmental and Maritime Hydraulic Laboratory (LIam) and leader of the Coastal Research Group. He completed his PhD at the University of "Roma Tre", with a thesis related to the impulse waves generated by landslide. Then, he spent several years at the early stage of his career at the University of Rome "Tor Vergata", before moving to the University of L'Aquila. He carries out research work in collaboration with both Italian and international research groups, by means of theoretical, numerical and experimental approaches in the fields of coastal engineering, harbor engineering and landslide generated tsunami waves. He has a large amount of experience in hydraulic laboratory tests in 2D wave flumes and, partially, in 3D wave tanks. His main research topics may be summarized as follows: the generation and propagation of landslide impulse generated waves, the real time detection of tsunamis, mathematical and experimental modeling of coastal processes, mathematical and experimental modeling of hydraulic and maritime structures, the development of wave energy converters, mathematical modeling of environmental impacts related to marine sediments handling, coastal risk and management, modeling of storm surge.

Donald F. Hayes is a Research Environmental Engineer in the Environmental Laboratory of the US Army Corps of Engineers' Engineer Research and Development Center (ERDC) in Vicksburg, MS. He earned a PhD in Civil Engineering from Colorado State University with an emphasis in Environmental Engineering and Water Resources Planning and Management. His research interests include environmental impacts associated with dredging and sediment management, particularly contaminated sediment management, wetland restoration, systems applications in water resources management, and water quality modeling. He has published widely and holds multiple patents. Dr. Hayes has extensive consulting and expert witness experience. He is a registered Professional Engineer, Diplomate of the American Academy of Environmental Engineers, Fellow of the American Society of Civil Engineers, Director of the Western Dredging Association, and editor of the Journal of Dredging Engineering.

Davide Pasquali is a researcher of Maritime and Hydraulic Structures at the Department of Civil, Construction-Architectural and Environmental Engineering of the University of L'Aquila (Italy). He is part of the Coastal Research Group at the same university. He completed his PhD at the University of L'Aquila, with a thesis related to the hindcasting and forecasting of storm surge. He has a long research experience in Hydraulic Laboratory Tests. His main research topics may be summarized as follows: hindcast and forecast of storm surge, development of wave energy converters, wave resource and availability assessments, mathematical modeling of environmental impacts related to marine sediments handling, mathematical and experimental modeling of coastal processes, and hydraulic and maritime structures.

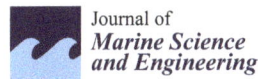

Editorial

Marine Sediments: Processes, Transport and Environmental Aspects

Marcello Di Risio [1], Donald F. Hayes [2] and Davide Pasquali [1,*]

1. Environmental and Maritime Hydraulic Laboratory (LIam), Department of Civil, Construction-Architectural and Environmental Engineering (DICEAA), University of L'Aquila, P.le Pontieri, 1, Monteluco di Roio, 67040 L'Aquila, Italy; marcello.dirisio@univaq.it
2. U.S. Army Engineer Research and Development Center, Engineer Research and Development Center, Environmental Laboratory, 3909 Halls Ferry Road, Vicksburg, MS 39180-6199, USA; Donald.F.Hayes@usace.army.mil
* Correspondence: davide.pasquali@univaq.it

Received: 23 March 2020; Accepted: 26 March 2020; Published: 2 April 2020

Keywords: marine sediment; contaminated sediment management; coastal sediment transport; harbor siltation; dredging; water quality; coastal engineering; coastal defence system; mathematical modelling; engineering practice

---

1. Introduction

In recent years, increasing attention has been paid to water quality and environmental aspects related to sediment transport driven by both ambient forcing and human activities. The increasing attention paid to this wide topic is also exacerbated by the exploitation of the coastal zone for economic, touristic and social reasons (e.g., [1]). Indeed, estuarine, coastal, and harbor areas often undergo operations that temporarily increase sediment transport, e.g., to nourish beaches, to maintain navigation channels, and to remove contaminated sediment primarily to support their use. For example, beach maintenance is required to counteract erosion processes that degrade beach quality. Sand has to be dredged and moved to nourish beaches (e.g., [2]). Moreover, harbor areas and navigation channels require maintenance dredging (e.g., [3]) to allow the regular circulation of the vessels and, in some cases, to remove contaminated sediments.

Particular interest is focused on water quality and environmental aspects related to sediment transport driven by anthropogenic activities. The impact of these activities on water quality (e.g., [4]) and on the human health is a significant public concern (e.g., [5]). Therefore, it is important to have reliable tools able to provide a realistic forecasts of the plume dispersion (e.g., [6–9]). Hence, much research is needed related to the sediment processes, transport, and related environmental aspects of marine sediments.

The aim of this Special Issue is to collect novel research results to improve knowledge and to propose new tools in this field. The issue collected five papers that cover different aspects of coastal and ocean engineering, chemical oceanography, geology, and geomorphology using different approaches and instruments. Some of the studies used numerical models [10,11], others acquired and analyzed field data regarding chemical [12] or geomorphological aspects of the ocean [13] while Lisi et al. [14] suggested a mathematical modeling framework to analyze the effects of sediment handling operations.

The core aspects of each paper are synthesized in the following section.

2. Papers Details

Hu et al. [10] investigate the important aspect of spillover of sediments due to the occurrence of typical tidal processes. The study was devoted to analyzing the case study of the Yangtze River's Estuary. They proposed a 2D numerical model based on the resolution of the depth-averaged 2D shallow water equations. The model is able to simulate the tidal flow, the sediment transport, and eventually the bed evolution in the estuary. Moreover, it allows giving a quantitative estimation regarding the spillover of water and sediment in the analyzed river. They used a high-resolution unstructured grid covering a great part of the river estuary (more that 600 km) to reproduce the Yangtze Estuary. The validation of the results against field data showed the good performances of the model in reproducing tidal levels, sediment concentration, and depth-averaged velocity.

Botsou et al. [12] analyzed the aspects related to metals' mobility in the water column, focusing their attention on Antinioti Lagoon and Corfu Island. In particular, they investigated the processes responsible for the mobility of metals both in and beyond the transitional fresh–saline water interface. They acquired water samples in two sampling campaigns, as well as surface and core sediments during only the first and second campaigns, respectively. These data were analyzed by means of trace metal analysis. They also performed a statistical analysis to evaluate the significant differences in terms of metal concentrations.

Johnson et al. [13] investigated the role of hurricanes on the modification of the rocky coastline in the Gulf of California, in the Ensenada Almeja in particular. They acquired field data to classify the weight and density of the rocks and performed a study on the hydrodynamic forces needed to move the largest boulders in the site. Geological and lithological characterization of the study area was performed by the authors. Moreover, they collected an aerial photo to map the coastal boulder bed of Ensenada Almeja. In this way, boulder shapes and sizes were evaluated and correlated with the wave heights required to lift the rocks from the bedrock.

Lisi et al. [14] proposed an integrated modeling approach useful for the simulation of sediment dispersion in several types of coastal areas (i.e., semi-enclosed basins and off-shore areas). At first, the attention is focused on the definition of sediment resuspension sources. Then, a definition of the level of accuracy that should be required in modeling activities is proposed. Moreover, they proposed a wide spectrum of possible modeling approaches that could be used by contractors and controlling authorities for scheduling and performing sediment handling activities, giving also a methodological approach useful to read and interpret the numerical results. They also underlined the importance of a modeling–monitoring feedback system.

Kuznetsova and Saprykina [11] analyzed how the beach profile is influenced by the location of underwater bars. They performed this study by using a numerical model with attention paid to the time scale of a given storm. The experiments were numerical; however, they used realistic boundary conditions and wave climate. The results reveal a direct correlation between the location of the underwater bar and the shoreline. Moreover, they found an inverse correlation between the retreat of the shoreline and low-frequency wave heights occurring at the coast.

Author Contributions: All authors contributed equally to this manuscript. All authors have read and agreed to the published version of the manuscript.

Funding: This research received no external funding.

Acknowledgments: We want to express our sincere thankfulness to all the authors and the reviewers.

Conflicts of Interest: The authors declare no conflict of interest.

References

1. Di Risio, M.; Bruschi, A.; Lisi, I.; Pesarino, V.; Pasquali, D. Comparative analysis of coastal flooding vulnerability and hazard assessment at national scale. *J. Mar. Sci. Eng.* **2017**, *5*, 51. [CrossRef]
2. Di Risio, M.; Lisi, I.; Beltrami, G.; De Girolamo, P. Physical modeling of the cross-shore short-term evolution of protected and unprotected beach nourishments. *Ocean Eng.* **2010**, *37*, 777–789. [CrossRef]
3. Nichols, M.M.; Howard-Strobel, M.M. Evolution of an urban estuarine harbor: Norfolk, Virginia. *J. Coast. Res.* **1991**, *7*, 745–757.

4. Bridges, T.S.; Ells, S.; Hayes, D.; Mount, D.; Nadeau, S.C.; Palermo, M.R.; Patmont, C.; Schroeder, P. *The Four rs of Environmental Dredging: Resuspension, Release, Residual, and Risk*; Technical Report; Engineer Research and Development Center: Vicksburg, MS, USA, 2008.
5. Feola, A.; Lisi, I.; Venti, F.; Salmeri, A.; Pedroncini, A.; Romano, E. A methodological modelling approach to assess the potential environmental impacts of dredging activities. In Proceedings of the Dredging Dredging Days, Innovative Dredging Solutions for Ports, Rotterdam The Netherlands, 5–6 November 2015.
6. Je, C.H.; Hayes, D.F. Development of a two-dimensional analytical model for predicting toxic sediment plumes due to environmental dredging operations. *J. Environ. Sci. Heal. Part A* **2004**, *39*, 1935–1947. [CrossRef] [PubMed]
7. Je, C.; Hayes, D.F.; Kim, K.S. Simulation of resuspended sediments resulting from dredging operations by a numerical flocculent transport model. *Chemosphere* **2007**, *70*, 187–195. [CrossRef] [PubMed]
8. Shao, D.; Gao, W.; Purnama, A.; Guo, J. Modeling dredging-induced turbidity plumes in the far field under oscillatory tidal currents. *J. Waterw. Port Coast. Ocean Eng.* **2017**, *143*, 06016007. [CrossRef]
9. Di Risio, M.; Pasquali, D.; Lisi, I.; Romano, A.; Gabellini, M.; De Girolamo, P. An analytical model for preliminary assessment of dredging-induced sediment plume of far-field evolution for spatial non homogeneous and time varying resuspension sources. *Coast. Eng.* **2017**, *127*, 106–118. [CrossRef]
10. Hu, D.; Wang, M.; Yao, S.; Jin, Z. Study on the Spillover of Sediment during Typical Tidal Processes in the Yangtze Estuary Using a High-Resolution Numerical Model. *J. Mar. Sci. Eng.* **2019**, *7*, 390. [CrossRef]
11. Kuznetsova, O.; Saprykina, Y. Influence of underwater bar location on cross-shore sediment transport in the coastal zone. *J. Mar. Sci. Eng.* **2019**, *7*, 55. [CrossRef]
12. Botsou, F.; Karageorgis, A.P.; Paraskevopoulou, V.; Dassenakis, M.; Scoullos, M. Critical Processes of Trace Metals Mobility in Transitional Waters: Implications from the Remote, Antinioti Lagoon, Corfu Island, Greece. *J. Mar. Sci. Eng.* **2019**, *7*, 307. [CrossRef]
13. Johnson, M.E.; Guardado-France, R.; Johnson, E.M.; Ledesma-Vázquez, J. Geomorphology of a Holocene Hurricane Deposit Eroded from Rhyolite Sea Cliffs on Ensenada Almeja (Baja California Sur, Mexico). *J. Mar. Sci. Eng.* **2019**, *7*, 193. [CrossRef]
14. Lisi, I.; Feola, A.; Bruschi, A.; Pedroncini, A.; Pasquali, D.; Di Risio, M. Mathematical Modeling Framework of Physical Effects Induced by Sediments Handling Operations in Marine and Coastal Areas. *J. Mar. Sci. Eng.* **2019**, *7*, 149. [CrossRef]

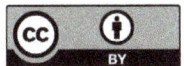

© 2020 by the authors. Licensee MDPI, Basel, Switzerland. This article is an open access article distributed under the terms and conditions of the Creative Commons Attribution (CC BY) license (http://creativecommons.org/licenses/by/4.0/).

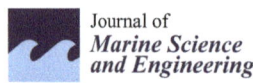

Article

Study on the Spillover of Sediment during Typical Tidal Processes in the Yangtze Estuary Using a High-Resolution Numerical Model

Dechao Hu [1], Min Wang [2], Shiming Yao [2] and Zhongwu Jin [2,*]

1 School of Hydropower and Information Engineering, Huazhong University of Science and Technology, Wuhan 430074, China; hudc04@foxmail.com
2 Department of River Engineering, Yangtze River Scientific Research Institute, Wuhan 430010, China; jss9871@vip.163.com (M.W.); yzhshymq@163.com (S.Y.)
* Correspondence: zhongwujin@163.com; Tel.: +86-027-8282-9873

Received: 16 August 2019; Accepted: 24 October 2019; Published: 1 November 2019

Abstract: Because of special morphologies and complex runoff–tide interactions, the landward floodtide flows in Yangtze Estuary are observed to spill over from the North to the South Branches, carrying a lot of sediment. To quantitatively clarify the spillover problem, a two-dimensional numerical model using a high-resolution channel-refined unstructured grid is developed for the entire Yangtze Estuary from Datong to river mouths (620 km) and part of the East Sea. The developed model ensures a good description of the river-coast-ocean coupling, the irregular boundaries, and local river regimes in the Yangtze Estuary. In tests, the simulated histories of the tidal level, depth-averaged velocity, and sediment concentration agree well with field data. The spillover of sediment in the Yangtze Estuary is studied using the condition of a spring and a neap tide in dry seasons. For a representative cross-section in the upper reach of the North Branch (QLG), the difference of the cross-sectional sediment flux (*CSSF*) between floodtide and ebbtide durations is 43.85–11.26 × 10^4 t/day, accounting for 37.5–34.9% of the landward floodtide *CSSF*. The mechanics of sediment spillover in Yangtze Estuary are clarified in terms of a successive process comprising the source, transport, and drainage of the spillover sediment.

Keywords: Yangtze estuary; tidal flows; sediment transport; sediment spillover; morphological dynamics; high-resolution; numerical model

1. Introduction

The Yangtze Estuary is a large-scale shallow water system characterized by three-level bifurcations (North and South Branches, North and South Channels, North and South Passages) and has four outlets into the East Sea (see in Figures 1 and 2). Significant runoff from the Yangtze River (about 9000 × 10^8 m^3/year) and periodical tides from the ocean meet in the estuary and interact with each other, leading to complicated hydrodynamics and sediment transport. The landward floodtide flow often spills over from the North to the South Branches, carrying a lot of sediment. The estuarine circulations of water and sediment fluxes, characterized by the spillover of water and sediment, play an important role in shaping the morphology of the Yangtze Estuary [1–5].

The spillover of water and sediment in the Yangtze Estuary is very complex because of the special morphology and the complex runoff-tide interactions. First, the spillover happens in a three-level branching estuary, where the exchanges of water and sediment are complex between different branches of the branching Yangtze Estuary. Second, the North Branch of the Yangtze Estuary is characterized by a special morphology [5]. The upper reach is narrow and almost orthogonal to the South Branch, preventing upstream inflows from entering during ebbtides. The lower and tail reaches are trumpet-shaped with a wide outlet, in favor of accommodating a great deal of landward tidal flows during floodtides. Third, the river, the coast, and the ocean in the Yangtze Estuary are closely related, where the bidirectional flows inside the estuary evolve gradually into clockwise irregular rotational tidal flows in offshore regions (under the influence of runoff-tide interactions, rapidly varying topographies and complex solid boundaries in coastal areas). As a result, it is difficult to study the spillover problem of water and sediment in the Yangtze Estuary. Moreover, because of limitations of field data and methods (the details will be introduced in the following paragraphs), quantitative studies on the spillover of sediment from the North to the South Branches in the Yangtze Estuary have not been reported. The quantitative knowledge on the spillover of sediment in the Yangtze Estuary is currently quite limited.

On the other hand, surrounded by the most developed regions of China (Shanghai city and Jiangsu Province), the Yangtze Estuary has seen extensive launching of flood-defense, water-resource, reclamation, and navigation projects because of requirements for the development of cities. It is generally necessary to check the reasonability of the designed constructions before launching a project. The influences of a project on the estuarine environment (e.g., the tidal flow, sediment transport, and long-term riverbed evolutions) should also be evaluated to clarify its possible negative side and for corresponding preventions. Under the influence of the spillover of water and sediment, figuring out the aforementioned issues of a project in the branching Yangtze Estuary is challenging. As a result, it is important to have extensive knowledge of the horizontal circulations of water-sediment fluxes in the Yangtze Estuary, which will provide a guide and a support for the design of constructions in real applications.

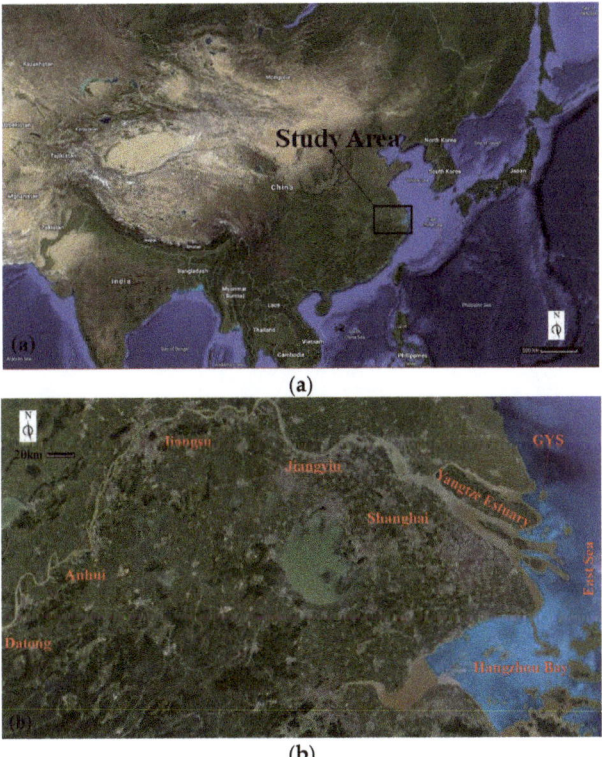

Figure 1. The location of the Yangtze Estuary and the study area (a Google Map diagram showing the geographical features of the location). (**a**) Location; (**b**) Tidal reaches and estuary.

The tidal flows and sediment transport in the Yangtze Estuary are often studied by analyzing field data using the physical model or adopting the numerical models. However, the knowledge based on the analysis of topographical and hydrological data is often limited by space–time resolutions of the field data of sediment transport. Existing studies of analysis are often only carried out for local reaches or parts of cross-sections in some branches of the Yangtze Estuary, e.g., the sediment transport rate along the streamline of main-flow channels [1,2,6]. Scale models are expensive to build and operate. As an effective and less expensive method, many numerical models have gradually become the most widely used method in studying estuarine hydrodynamics and sediment transport due to continuous improvements in computers and numerical schemes.

Two-dimensional (2D) or three-dimensional (3D) numerical models applied to the Yangtze Estuary should meet the multiple requirements for computational accuracy and efficiency. First, to get a full description of river-coast-ocean coupling, the upstream tidal reach, the entire Yangtze Estuary and part of the East Sea are included in a single model. The computational domain of the entire Yangtze Estuary (from Datong to seaward contours of −4 m) is 84.4×10^8 m^2, as shown in Figure 2. Second, the computational grid should be fine enough to describe well the local river regimes in the Yangtze Estuary and simulate the estuarine mesoscale structures and transport process correctly [7,8]. Corresponding to fine grids, a small time step of 1–2 min is often required to ensure the stability and accuracy in simulating the fully unsteady flows and sediment transport. Third, simulations of long-term tidal flows, sediment transport, and riverbed evolution are often required in studies of the morphological dynamics. When the domain of the entire Yangtze Estuary is divided using a high-resolution grid, a huge computational cost is required. These requirements challenge almost all existing 2D or 3D numerical models [9]. As a result, in real applications of the Yangtze Estuary, researchers often have to use coarse grids, establish local models [10–12], or adopt simplified methods, such as the method of the morphological scale factor [13,14].

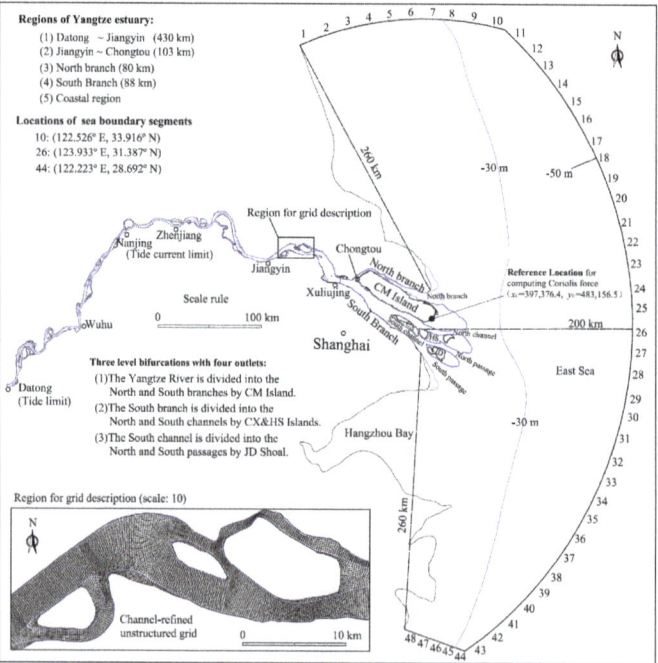

Figure 2. Description of the bound, the three-level bifurcations and the strong river-coast-sea coupling in Yangtze Estuary (computational domain and grid are also given).

In this paper, an efficient 2D numerical model is developed to simulate the tidal flow, sediment transport, and riverbed evolution in the Yangtze Estuary using a high-resolution channel-refined unstructured grid. The model is then applied to a quantitative study on the mechanics of the spillover of water and sediment in the Yangtze Estuary.

2. Numerical Formulation

The governing equations, computational grids, and numerical schemes of the hydrodynamic model (HDM) and the sediment transport model (STM) are introduced.

2.1. Governing Equations

Depth-averaged 2D shallow water equations (SWEs), with Coriolis terms, are used as the governing equations for the HDM, which are given by

$$\frac{\partial \eta}{\partial t} + \frac{\partial (hu)}{\partial x} + \frac{\partial (hv)}{\partial y} = 0 \tag{1}$$

$$\frac{\partial u}{\partial t} + u\frac{\partial u}{\partial x} + v\frac{\partial u}{\partial y} = fv - g\frac{\partial \eta}{\partial x} + \frac{\tau_{sx}}{\rho h} - g\frac{n_m^2 u \sqrt{u^2 + v^2}}{h^{4/3}} + v_t\left(\frac{\partial^2 u}{\partial x^2} + \frac{\partial^2 u}{\partial y^2}\right) \tag{2a}$$

$$\frac{\partial v}{\partial t} + u\frac{\partial v}{\partial x} + v\frac{\partial v}{\partial y} = -fu - g\frac{\partial \eta}{\partial y} + \frac{\tau_{sy}}{\rho h} - g\frac{n_m^2 v \sqrt{u^2 + v^2}}{h^{4/3}} + v_t\left(\frac{\partial^2 v}{\partial x^2} + \frac{\partial^2 v}{\partial y^2}\right) \tag{2b}$$

where $h(x, y, t)$ is the water depth, (m); $u(x, y, t)$ and $v(x, y, t)$ are the components of depth-averaged velocity in the horizontally in the x- and y-directions, respectively, (m/s); t is the time, (s); g is the gravitational acceleration, (m/s^2); $\eta(x, y, t)$ is the water level measured from an undisturbed reference water surface, (m); v_t is the coefficient of the horizontal eddy viscosity, (m^2/s); f is Coriolis factor; n_m is Manning's roughness coefficient, (m$^{-1/3}$ s); ρ is the water density, (kg/m^3); and τ_{sx} and τ_{sy} are the wind stress in the x- and y-directions, respectively, (N/m^2).

The above equations construct a set of equations for u, v and η. Their forms are invariable in the rotating frame of unstructured grids. The wind stress is imposed as per [12,13]. For a given location (x, y) of the Yangtze Estuary, the Coriolis factor f is given by

$$f = 2\Omega \sin\left(\frac{\pi}{180}\phi + \frac{y - y_c}{6357.0 \times 1000}\right) \tag{3}$$

where Ω (7.29 × 10^{-5} rad/s) is the angular velocity of rotation of the Earth; ϕ (31.38724°) is the latitude of the reference location (x_c, y_c) which is shown in Figure 2.

The annual bed-load quantity transported through the outlets of the Yangtze Estuary is about 500–1000 × 10^4 tons, accounting for 1–2% of the total sediment load [15]. The bed-load transport therefore contributes little to the horizontal circulations of global water–sediment fluxes in the Yangtze Estuary, and is not solved by the present model. The suspended sediment is regarded to be nonuniform and is described by a fraction method. The vertically averaged 2D advection–diffusion equation, with a source term describing sediment exchange between flow and riverbed, is used to describe the transport of nonuniform suspended load:

$$\frac{\partial (hC_k)}{\partial t} + \frac{\partial (uhC_k)}{\partial x} + \frac{\partial (vhC_k)}{\partial y} = \frac{v_t}{\sigma_c}\left[\frac{\partial^2 (hC_k)}{\partial x^2} + \frac{\partial^2 (hC_k)}{\partial y^2}\right] + \alpha w_{sk}(S_{*k} - C_k) \tag{4}$$

where k is the index of the sediment fraction, $k = 1, 2, \ldots, N_s$ (N_s is the number of fractions); C_k and S_{*k} = sediment concentration and the sediment-carrying capacity of flows for the k_{th} fraction of the nonuniform suspended load, respectively, kg/m^3; w_{sk} = settling velocity of sediment particles for the k_{th} fraction of the suspended load, m/s; α = sediment recovery coefficient, which is set to 1.0 and 0.25, respectively, in case of erosion and deposition [16].

According to particle size and physical/chemical property, the nonuniform sediment is divided into four fractions. The size ranges of fractions 1–4 are, sequentially, 0–0.031, 0.031–0.125, 0.125–0.5, and >0.5 mm. In real applications, researchers often determined the settling velocity (w_s) of the fine particles according to field data, experiments or their experience [11,12,17–20]. In the present model, the w_s of fraction 1 is set according to field data in the Yangtze Estuary, while the primitive settling velocity is directly used for other fractions.

Zhang's formula [21], which is widely used in evaluating the sediment-carrying capacity of flows in real applications, is used in our model and given by

$$S_{*k} = K\left[U^3/(ghw_{sk})\right]^m \tag{5}$$

where U is a vertically averaged velocity ($U = \sqrt{u^2 + v^2}$); m is an exponent and set to 0.92 in our model; K is sediment-carrying coefficient and determined by calibrations with field data. In the model, Zhang's formula [21], with the help of the method in [22], is used to determine the fractional sediment-carrying capacities of flows for the nonuniform sediment.

Corresponding to Equation (4), riverbed deformation induced by the transport of the k_{th} fraction of the nonuniform suspended load is described by

$$\rho' \frac{\partial z_{bk}}{\partial t} = \alpha w_{sk}(C_k - S_{*k}) \tag{6}$$

where z_{bk} = riverbed deformation caused by the k_{th} fraction sediment, m; ρ' = dry density of bed materials, kg/m³. The gradation state of the bed materials is also updated using the method of [22].

The coefficient of Manning's roughness, n_m, in the HDM and the coefficient of the sediment-carrying capacity, K, in the STM are determined by calibration tests with field data. Because the Yangtze Estuary is large and includes various regions with different characteristics of flows and sediment transports (e.g., river reach, tidal reach, coast sea area, and sea region), non-constant model parameters are used in different regions.

2.2. Computational Grid and Model Formulation

2.2.1. Computational Grid

The computational domain is divided up by a set of non-overlapping triangles or convex quadrangles. A CD staggered grid of variable arrangement [23] is used. The horizontal velocity components, u and v, are defined at side (cell face) centers, while the water level, η, and the scalar concentration, C, are defined at element centroids. The notations ne, np, and ns are respectively used to denote the number of elements (cells), nodes, and sides of the unstructured grid. For the sake of convenience, the notations associated with the unstructured grid are introduced as follows:

(1) $i34(i)$ is the number of nodes/sides of cell i; $j(i,l)$ is the sides of cell i, where $l = 1, 2, \ldots, i34(i)$; P_i is the area of cell i; (2) $i(j,l)$ are two cells that share side j, where $l = 1, 2$; δ_j is the distance between two adjacent cell centroids that are separated by side j; L_j is the length of side j; (3) $s_{i,l}$ is a sign function associated with the orientation of the normal velocity defined on side l of cell i. Specifically, $s_{i,l} = 1/-1$ if a positive velocity on side l of cell i corresponds to outflow/inflow (of cell i).

2.2.2. Numerical Discretizations

The adopted HDM uses a θ semi-implicit formulation [24–26], while finite-volume and finite-difference methods are combined. Momentum equations are solved within a finite-difference framework and using operator-splitting techniques. The θ semi-implicit method is used to advance the time stepping. Correspondingly, the gradient of the free-surface elevation is discretized into explicit and implicit parts. A point-wise Eulerian-Lagrangian method (ELM), using the multistep backward

Euler technique [23,27], is used to solve the advection term. The horizontal diffusion term is discretized using an explicit center-difference method.

When the advection term is solved by the ELM, the velocities are updated at once and are denoted by u_{bt} and v_{bt}. The horizontal momentum equations in the local horizontal x-, y-directions of unstructured grids are then discretized as follows (at side j)

$$\left(1 + \Delta t g n_m^2 \frac{\sqrt{u_{bt,j}^{n}{}^2 + v_{bt,j}^{n}{}^2}}{h_j^{n4/3}}\right) u^{n+1} = u_{bt,j}^n - \Delta t g \left[(1-\theta) \frac{\eta_{i(j,2)}^n - \eta_{i(j,1)}^n}{\delta_j} + \theta \frac{\eta_{i(j,2)}^{n+1} - \eta_{i(j,1)}^{n+1}}{\delta_j}\right] + \Delta t E_X^n{}_j \quad (7a)$$

$$\left(1 + \Delta t g n_m^2 \frac{\sqrt{u_{bt,j}^{n}{}^2 + v_{bt,j}^{n}{}^2}}{h_j^{n4/3}}\right) v^{n+1} = v_{bt,j}^n - \Delta t g \left[(1-\theta) \frac{\eta_{ip(j,2)}^n - \eta_{ip(j,1)}^n}{L_j} + \theta \frac{\eta_{ip(j,2)}^{n+1} - \eta_{ip(j,1)}^{n+1}}{L_j}\right] + \Delta t E_Y^n{}_j \quad (7b)$$

where θ is the implicit factor and Δt the time step; superscripts "n" indicate the n-th time step; for simplicity, the explicitly discretized horizontal diffusion term is not expanded here; the riverbed friction is discretized using u_{bt} and v_{bt} to enhance computation stability. The explicitly discretized horizontal diffusion term is not expanded here for simplicity, and denoted by E_X and E_Y in x- and y-directions, respectively. The η at nodes is regarded as auxiliary variables, which are interpolated from water-level values of neighboring cells.

When explicit terms of the discretized momentum equations are incorporated, the unknowns (free-surface elevation η) emerge. Equation (7a,b) are then transformed into (at side j)

$$u_j^{n+1} = G_j^n / A_j^n - \theta g \Delta t \frac{\eta_{i(j,2)}^{n+1} - \eta_{i(j,1)}^{n+1}}{\delta_j} / A_j^n \quad (8a)$$

$$v_j^{n+1} = F_j^n / A_j^n - \theta g \Delta t \frac{\eta_{ip(j,2)}^{n+1} - \eta_{ip(j,1)}^{n+1}}{L_j} / A_j^n \quad (8b)$$

where $A_j^n = 1 + \Delta t g n_m^2 \sqrt{u_{bt_j}^{n}{}^2 + u_{bt_j}^{n}{}^2} / h_j^{n4/3}$; G_j^n, F_j^n are the incorporated explicit terms respectively in the horizontal x-, y-directions, $G_j^n = u_{bt,j}^n - \Delta t g (1-\theta) \frac{\eta_{i(j,2)}^n - \eta_{i(j,1)}^n}{\delta_j} + \Delta t E_X^n{}_j$, $F_j^n = v_{bt,j}^n - \Delta t g (1-\theta) \frac{\eta_{ip(j,2)}^n - \eta_{ip(j,1)}^n}{L_j} + \Delta t E_Y^n{}_j$.

To achieve good mass conservation, the depth-integrated continuity equation, Equation (1), is discretized by the finite-volume method, which is given by (at cell i)

$$P_i \eta_i^{n+1} = P_i \eta_i^n - \theta \Delta t \sum_{l=1}^{i34(i)} s_{i,l} L_{j(i,l)} h_{j(i,l)}^n u_{j(i,l)}^{n+1} - (1-\theta) \Delta t \sum_{l=1}^{i34(i)} s_{i,l} L_{j(i,l)} h_{j(i,l)}^n u_{j(i,l)}^n \quad (9)$$

where l is the side index of cell i, and $l = 1, 2, \ldots, i34(i)$.

The velocity–pressure coupling is performed by substituting u_j^{n+1} and v_j^{n+1} of Equation (8a,b) into the discrete depth-integrated continuity equation. This substitution results in a wave propagation equation with cell water levels (η) as unknowns. Using the topology relations among the cells, the resulting discrete wave propagation equation is given by (at cell i)

$$\begin{aligned} P_i \eta_i^{n+1} + g \theta^2 \Delta t^2 \sum_{l=1}^{i34(i)} \frac{L_{j(i,l)}}{\delta_j} h_{j(i,l)}^n \left(\eta_i^{n+1} - \eta_{ic3(i,l)}^{n+1}\right) / A_{j(i,l)}^n \\ = P_i \eta_i^n - \theta \Delta t \sum_{l=1}^{i34(i)} s_{i,l} L_{j(i,l)} h_{j(i,l)}^n G_{j(i,l)}^n / A_{j(i,l)}^n - (1-\theta) \Delta t \sum_{l=1}^{i34(i)} s_{i,l} L_{j(i,l)} h_{j(i,l)}^n u_{j(i,l)}^n \end{aligned} \quad (10)$$

The HDM solves the vertically averaged 2D shallow water equations at three steps. First, all the explicit terms (advection, diffusion, riverbed friction, and the explicit part of free-surface gradients) in momentum equations are explicitly computed to obtain the provisional velocities. Second, the velocity-pressure coupling is performed by substituting the expressions of normal velocity components into the discrete continuity equation, where a wave propagation equation is constructed and solved to obtain new water levels. Third, a back substitution of the new water levels into the momentum equations is performed to get the final velocity field.

For each fraction of nonuniform sediment, one transport equation must be solved. The STM is advanced fully explicitly, and the transport equation is discretized as (for fraction k)

$$C_{k,i}^{n+1} = C_{k,bt,i}^{n+1} + \frac{\Delta t}{P_i h_i^n} \sum_{l=1}^{i34(i)} \left\{ s_{i,l} L_{j(i,l)} h_{j(i,l)}^n \left[\left(\frac{v_t}{\sigma_c}\right)_{j(i,l)}^n \frac{C_{k,i[j(i,l),2]}^n - C_{k,i[j(i,l),1]}^n}{\delta_{j(i,l)}} \right] \right\} + \frac{\Delta t}{h_i^n} \alpha_k w_{sk} \left(S_{*k}^n - C_k^n \right) \quad (11)$$

where Δt is the time step for the STM; C_{bt} is the solution to the advection subequation. The C_{bt} is calculated using a recently developed finite-volume ELM (FVELM) [28], where mass is conserved and large time steps (for which the Courant-Friedrichs-Lewy number (CFL) can be much greater than 1) are allowed.

For the FVELM, the geometrical computation which is common for each sediment fraction can be reused. When the most time-consuming parts (calculations of trajectories and interpolation weights) are avoided, only a relatively very small computation cost is added for solving each additional sediment fraction. Therefore, the FVELM allows constructing efficient algorithms for solving the transport of a large number of sediment fractions, and this property of the FVELM is defined as the multiscalar property. Benefiting from "allowing large time steps, parallelizable, multiscalar property", the FVELM is much more efficient than the traditional Eulerian advection schemes in solving the transport of nonuniform sediment with several fractions.

2.3. Parallelization of the Model Code

The HDM and STM can both be well parallelized. In the code of the model, the computation of one time step was implemented as a number of loops. Among these loops, the parallelizable ones were parallelized using loop-based parallelization and the open multiprocessing technique (OpenMP). In this study, a 16-core processor (Intel Xeon E5-2697a v4) and Intel C++ 14.0 formed the hardware and software environment. The runtime speedup, used as an indicator of how much faster the parallel code is than the sequential code, is defined by

$$Sp = T_1/T_{nc} \quad (12)$$

where Sp = speedup of a parallel run relative to a sequential run; T_1 = runtime of a sequential run using one working core; T_{nc} = runtime of a parallel run using n_c working cores.

3. Model Parameters and Tests

3.1. Computational Grid and Boundary Conditions

To get a full description of the river-coast-ocean coupling, the upstream tidal reach, the entire Yangtze Estuary and part of the East Sea are included in a single model. Station Datong (620 km upstream of the outlets), which is regarded as the tidal limit of the estuary and has routinely collected hydrological field data, was chosen as the upstream boundary. Seaward open boundaries are extended to deep-water (>50 m) regions, where a global tide model (GTM) [29] can provide an accurate history of astronomical tides. The eastern seaward open boundary is located around 124° E, with southern and northern boundaries being at 28.7° N and 33.9° N, respectively.

With three-level bifurcations and tens of islands or shoals, the Yangtze Estuary has complex river regimes [30]. The common resolution of bathymetry graphs, for an accurate description of the local river regimes of the Yangtze Estuary, is listed in Table 1. Coarse computational grids only describe an oversmoothed riverbed and are unable to correctly solve estuarine mesoscale structures [7] and transport process [8]. To ensure a good description of irregular boundaries and local river regimes, a channel-refined unstructured grid is used, whose grid scale (listed in Table 1) is approximately equal to the intervals between two neighboring survey points of the corresponding bathymetry graph. The main-flow channels in tidal reaches are covered by refined structured-like grids, with floodplains and inner islands covered by relatively coarse unstructured grids. There are 199,310 quad cells, and an example of the grid is given in Figure 2 (see Figure S1 for details).

Table 1. Grid scales of high-resolution unstructured grids in Yangtze Estuary.

Region	Length (km)	Area (km^2)	Resolution of Bathymetry Graph	Grid Scale (m × m)
Tidal reach	533	2066	1/10,000	200 × 80
North Branch	80	366	1/10,000	200 × 80–400 × 200
South Branch	88	1132	1/25,000	400 × 200
Coast region	-	8746	-	500–2000
East Sea	-	105,993	-	2000–5000

At the upstream boundary (see Figure 2), field data of discharges and sediment concentration at Station Datong were used to set the upstream boundary conditions. At downstream boundaries, the seaward open boundary is forced by semidiurnal tides. The time series of the tidal levels at the seaward boundary are predicted by the GTM developed in reference [29]. The seaward boundary is divided into 48 segments (see Figure 2), for each of which the tidal harmonic constants are, respectively, interpolated from a constituent database on a full global grid.

In calibration and validation tests of the HDM and the STM, the computational time step (Δt) is set to 90 s, and is equally divided into 9 sub time steps in the backtracking of the point-wise ELM.

3.2. Calibration and Validation Tests of HDM

Field data of spring neap tides during 6–16 December 2012 were used to calibrate parameters of the model and then validate its accuracy. In the hydrological survey, tidal levels were recorded at 14 fixed gauges from 6 December (the 340th day of 2012) to 16 December. The depth-averaged horizontal velocity was recorded from 8 December at 12:00 to 9 December at 21:00 for neap tides and from 14 December at 7:00 to 15 December at 13:00 for spring tides. Arrangements of the hydrological survey locations are shown in Figure 3. At the upstream boundary, the daily average river discharge at Station Datong gradually reduced from 22,000 to 18,700 m^3/s during 6–16 December 2012.

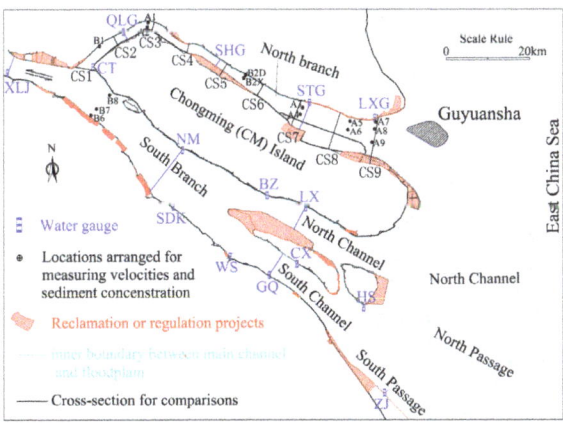

Figure 3. Arrangements of hydrology survey locations in Yangtze Estuary.

In the simulations, the time step of the HDM is set to 90 s, while nine sub steps are used in the backtracking of the ELM. For a simulation of free-surface flows, the initial condition has a significant effect on the simulation of unsteady flows. In our simulations, the initial condition was determined by a preliminary simulation.

Manning's roughness coefficient, n_m, was calibrated using the spring-tide condition from 14 December at 0:00 to 16 December at 0:00. The inflow discharge was set to 19,000 m³/s. The n_m of sub regions was adjusted so that the simulated tide-level histories would agree with field data. The n_m was then corrected slightly so that the simulated velocity histories would agree with field data at the same time. The n_m was finally calibrated as 0.022–0.021 from Station Datong to Jiangyin, 0.021–0.015 from Station Jiangyin to Xuliujing, and 0.014–0.011 for the North and South Branches. The n_m in the North and South Branches was similar to the values reported in previous research [31,32].

Using the aforementioned distribution of n_m, the histories of the simulated tidal levels and depth-averaged velocities were shown to agree well with field data. Generally, the mean absolute error in simulated tide levels was less than 0.15 m compared with the field data, while the mean absolute relative error in simulated velocity at survey positions was less than 10%. The accuracy of the model was then verified by simulating a full spring-neap tide process on 6–16 December 2012, and the simulation results are shown in Figures 4 and 5.

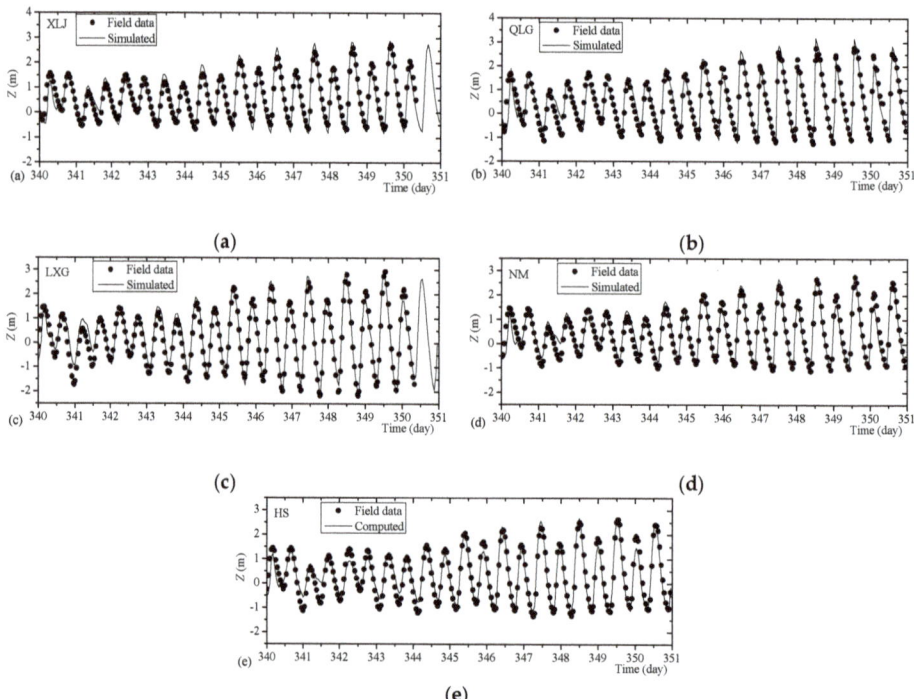

Figure 4. Comparisons of the simulated tide-level histories and field data. (**a**) at Station Xuliujing (XLJ), (**b**) at Station Qinglonggang (QLG), (**c**) at Station Lianxingang (LZG), (**d**) at Station Nanmen (NM), (**e**) at Station Hengsha (HS).

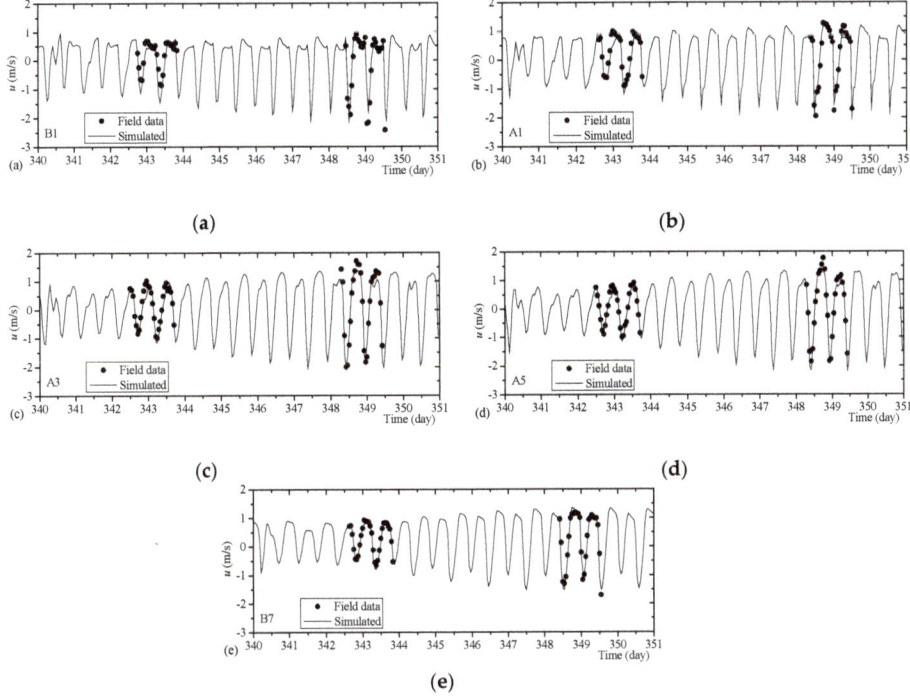

Figure 5. Comparisons of simulated histories of velocity with field data (negative velocity is landward velocity, which appears during the flood duration). (**a**) at Survey Point B1, (**b**) at Survey Point A1, (**c**) at Survey Point A3, (**d**) at Survey Point A5, (**e**) at Survey Point B7.

3.3. Calibration and Validation Tests of STM

The sediment-capacity coefficient, K, is also calibrated using the spring-tide condition from 2012/12/14 0:00 to 2012/12/16 0:00. At the upstream boundary, the river discharge and the sediment concentration are respectively 19,000 m^3/s and 0.112 kg/m^3. The parameter K is calibrated as 0.11–0.08 from Datong to Jiangyin, 0.07–0.04 from Jiangyin to Xuliujing, 0.05–0.02 for the North and the South Branches. Similar to the calibrated n_m, the calibrated K in coast sea regions of the Yangtze Estuary (0.07–0.02) also appears to be smaller than that of inland rivers (0.1–0.2), but approaches the values (about 0.07) reported by [32].

Using the aforementioned distribution of K, the STM is then verified by simulating a full spring neap tide process in the Yangtze Estuary on 6–16 December 2012. The histories of the simulated sediment concentration are generally observed to agree with field data, with minor amplitude errors (see Figure 6). The mean absolute relative errors in simulated sediment concentrations are generally less than 20%.

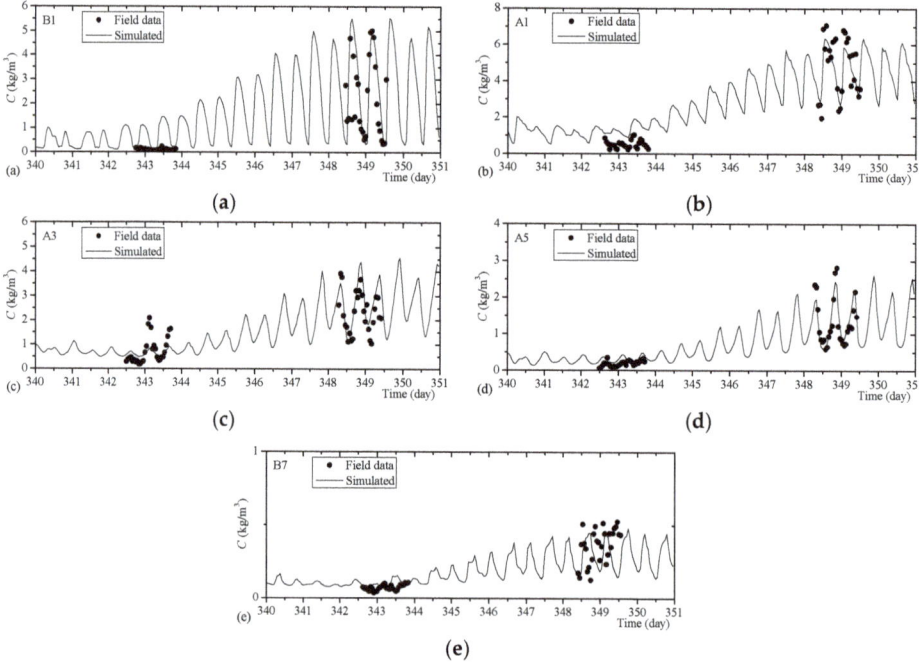

Figure 6. Comparisons of simulated sediment concentration histories and field data at survey locations. (**a**) at Survey Point B1, (**b**) at Survey Point A1, (**c**) at Survey Point A3, (**d**) at Survey Point A5, (**e**) at Survey Point B7.

On the one hand, Zhang's formula [21], used to evaluate the sediment-carrying capacity, does not involve an incipient velocity (the critical velocity at which sediment particles begin to move from a rest state). Hence, the sediment-carrying capacity calculated by Zhang's formula [21] is always sensitive to the velocity. In neap-tide periods, the calculated sediment-carrying capacity is closely related to the velocity of the flow, so the history of the simulated depth-averaged sediment concentration closely follows the tidal process. On the other hand, in the survey of field data, the depth-averaged sediment concentration is evaluated by using the measurements at different heights in a vertical line. However, during neap tides, the vertical distribution of sediment concentration is strongly nonuniform, and a great number of the transported sediment gathers in the bottom layers of the flow. The high concentration at bottom layers is often not caught or improperly measured because of the sensibility problem or the inaccurate vertical location of instruments. The vertical distribution of sediment concentration during spring-tide periods is much more uniform than that during neap-tide periods. It is easier to obtain the accurate sediment concentrations which can achieve a good representation of the value of the measured vertical line. This may explain that the data around day 343 (neap-tide periods) is poorly approximated and that around day 349 is fairly well reproduced in Figure 6a–c.

The topographical data of December 2011 and November 2013 are then employed to verify the module of bed evolution, where a simulation of 2-year unsteady flow, nonuniform sediment transport, and fluvial process from 2011/12/1 to 2013/11/30 in the Yangtze Estuary is carried out. During the 731 days, the total quantities of the runoff and the inflow sediment are respectively $17,947 \times 10^8$ m^3 and 2.854×10^8 tons. The daily river discharge and sediment concentration are imposed at the upstream boundary, while the seaward open boundaries are forced by tide levels of one-hour intervals. The measured topographical data in December 2011 is used to set the initial topography. The elevations of the nodes in the area of reclamations (or regulations) are modified to be consistent with the design, and the cells there are set to be non-erodible. Then, the model steps forward to November 2013 to get the final topography.

The simulated riverbeds at selected cross-sections of the North Branch (see Figure 3) are compared with those measured in November 2013, as shown in Figure 7. Generally, the simulated topographies at most cross-sections agree with field data. The reach, where cross-section CS5 is located, is narrowed by a project named "Xincun Sand regulation" which was launched during 2011–2013. In this reach, the flow is gathered, and the flow intensity is stronger than that in the original wider channel. As a result, the shallow sand is erased by the gathered flow after the time of the simulation. However, on the one hand, the disturbances from the projects of reclamations and regulations, launched in the North Branch during 2011–2013, may not be fully considered in the simulation. On the other hand, the present model does not have a module for simulating bank failures. Due to these disadvantages, the simulated riverbed evolutions at some cross-sections deviate from the field data. The North Branch experienced mild erosion form December 2012 to November 2013 in the simulation, which is consistent with the field. The erosion quantity of sediment is 5128.1×10^4 tons in the simulation, and has an error of +11.1% relative to field data.

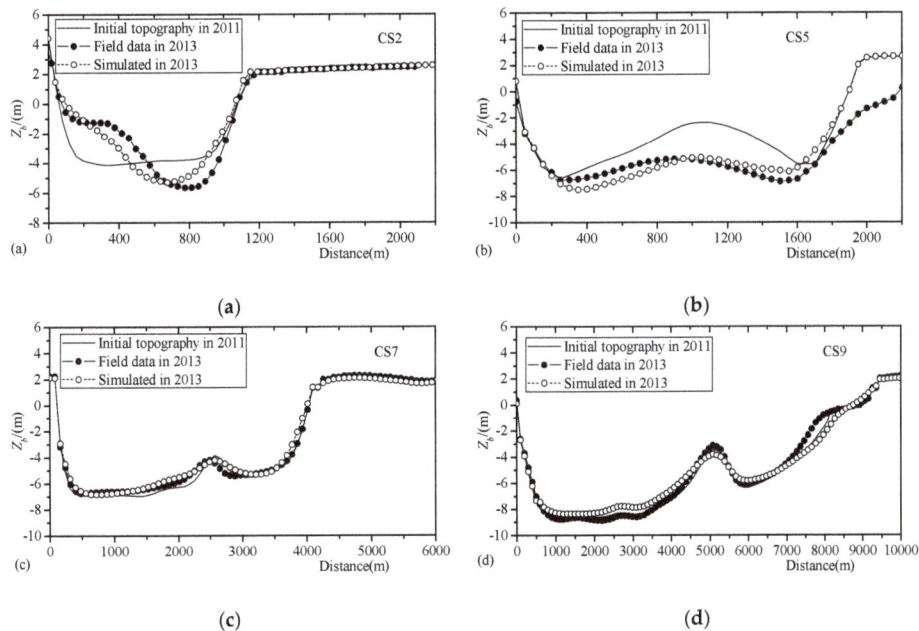

Figure 7. Comparisons of the simulated riverbed evolutions and field data at cross-sections. (**a**) at CS2, (**b**) at CS5, (**c**) at CS7, (**d**) at CS9.

3.4. Sensitivity Study of Model Parameters and Coefficients

Generally, the accuracy of a simulation may be sensitive to the variation of model parameters and coefficients, while simulation results vary with respect to them. The spring neap tide process in the Yangtze Estuary on 6–16 December 2012 is also used to perform the sensitivity studies of the main model parameters (e.g., Δt) and coefficients (e.g., n_m, and K).

First, the sensitivity study of time steps is performed. On the one hand, the use of a large time step means low time resolution of cell update, which will reduce the accuracy of the simulations of strongly unsteady tidal flows, such as those in the Yangtze Estuary. On the other hand, the ELM used in the current model becomes very dissipative at small time steps, per [27,33,34]. According to the tests of real shallow water systems in [25,26,28], the time step of the current model is suggested to be equal to or larger than 60 s, under a grid of moderate scale. Hence, the model is tested here on gradually reduced time steps which are sequentially 60, 75, 90, 100, and 120 s, to clarify the influence of time steps on the accuracy of solutions. Correspondingly, the number of substeps for the ELM backtracking (N_{bt}) is, respectively, set to 6, 8, 9, 10, and 12.

Under different time steps, the histories of the simulated tide level, survey-point velocity, and sediment concentration are shown in Figure 8, respectively (taking Station QLG and Survey Point A1 as examples). In a simulation of the adopted spring neap tide process, the mean absolute error in simulated tide levels is calculated to be 0.01–0.02 m, the mean absolute error in simulated survey-point velocities is 0.019–0.035 m/s, and the mean absolute error in simulated survey-point sediment concentrations is 2.8–3.5%, based on the simulated histories using different $\Delta t s$. Although minor differences are observed in the results of simulations using different time steps, the accuracies of the HDM and the STM are both stable with respect to the time step. The suggested time step (90 s) is revealed to be proper.

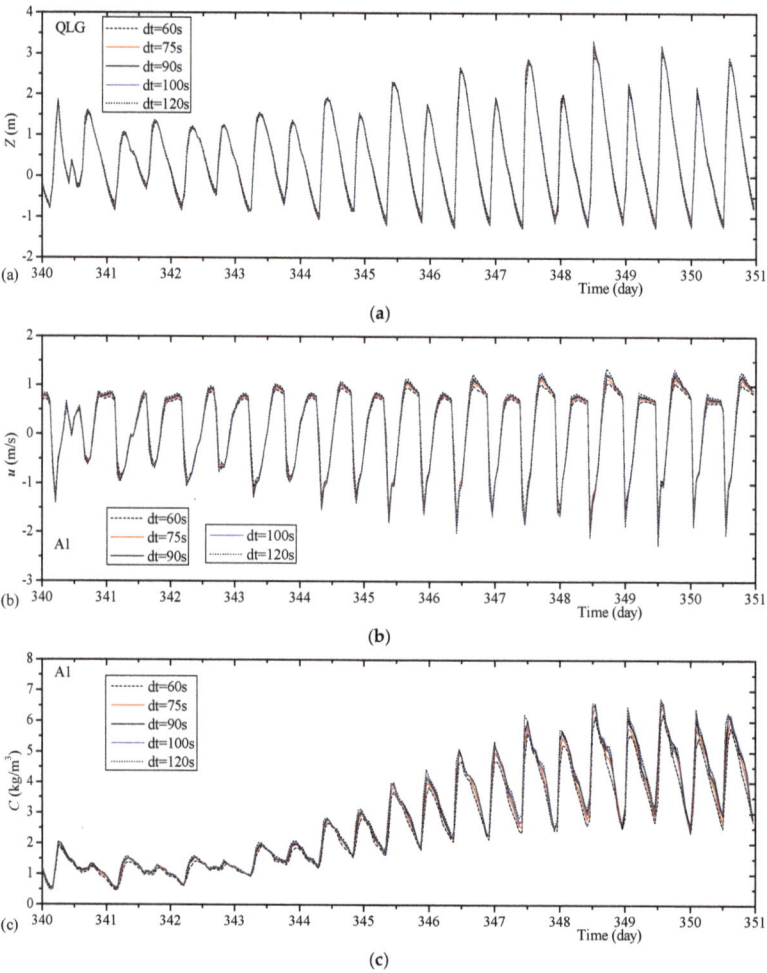

Figure 8. Comparisons of the simulated histories and field data. (**a**) Tide-level histories at Station Qinglonggang (QLG), (**b**) velocity histories at Survey Point A1, and (**c**) sediment concentration histories at Survey Point A1.

Second, the sensitivity study of the coefficient of Manning's roughness (n_m) is performed by changing the n_m in the North and the South Branches which are considered as the most important regions in this case study. The distribution of the n_m, obtained by the calibration test, is taken as the reference and is denoted by "original friction (nm)". The tests, with the n_m being reduced (−0.001) and increased (+0.001), are denoted by "nm −0.001" and "nm +0.001", respectively.

Under different n_m, the histories of the simulated tide level and survey-point velocity are, respectively, shown in Figure 9 (taking Station QLG and Survey Point A1 as examples). It is found that the smaller the n_m of the North and South Branches are, the stronger the landward floodtide flow in these reaches will be (characterized by higher tidal levels and large velocities). It is obvious that the variation of water levels with respect to the n_m is just opposite for the estuary tidal flows and for the inland river flows. The variation of the peak water level in Station QLG is +0.15 m when the n_m is reduced by 0.001, and is −0.04 m when the n_m is increased by 0.001. The variation of the peak velocity in Survey Point A1 is +0.12 m/s when the n_m is reduced by 0.001, and is −0.25 m/s when the n_m is increased by 0.001.

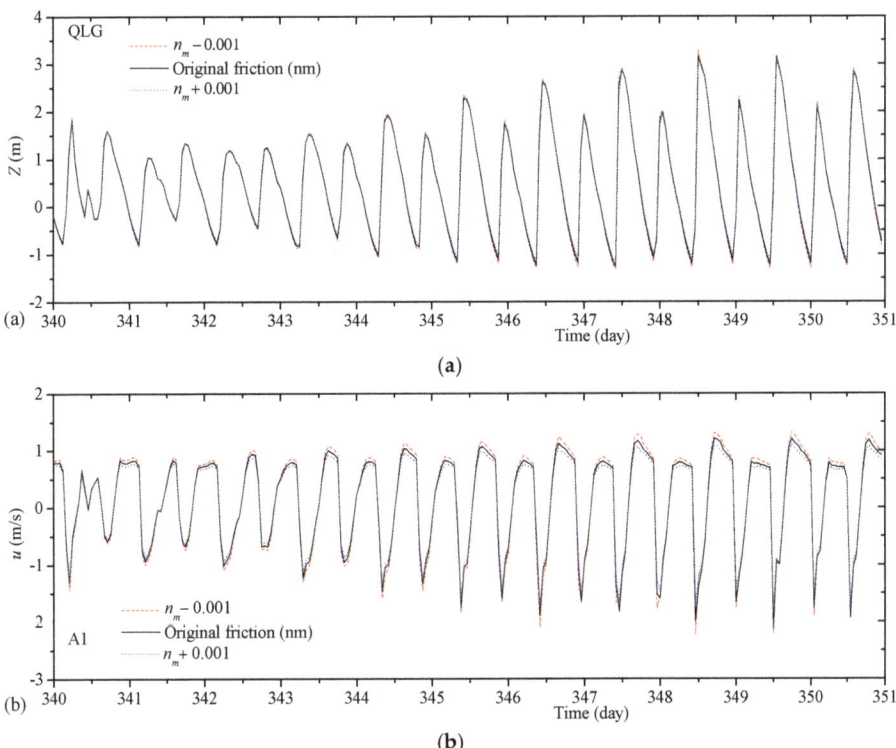

Figure 9. Comparisons of the simulated histories and field data. (**a**) Tide-level histories at Station Qinglonggang (QLG) and (**b**) velocity histories at Survey Point A1.

Third, the sensitivity study of the coefficient of sediment-carrying capacity (K) is performed by changing the K in the North and South Branches, which are considered as the most important regions in this case study. The distribution of the K, obtained by the calibration test, is taken as the reference and is denoted by "original coefficient". The tests, with the K being reduced (−0.002) and increased (+0.002), are denoted by "K −0.002" and "K +0.002", respectively.

Under different K, the histories of the simulated sediment concentration are shown in Figure 10 (taking Survey Point A1 as an example). It is found that the simulated sediment concentration increases with respect to K. The variation of the sediment concentration in Survey Point A1 is -0.33 kg/m^3 when the K is reduced by 0.002, and is $+0.25$ kg/m^3 when the K is increased by 0.002.

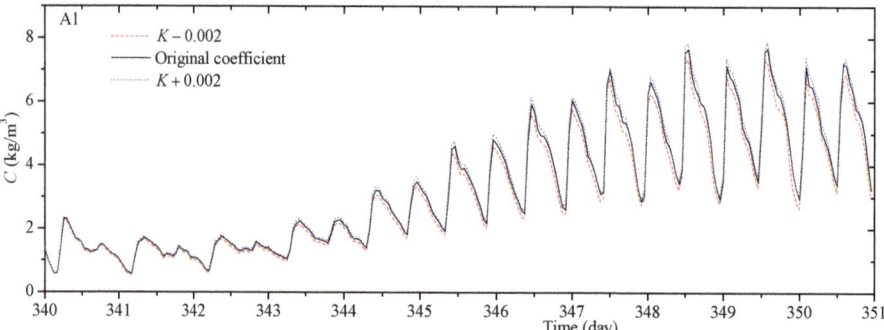

Figure 10. Comparisons of the histories of the simulated sediment concentration and field data (at Survey Point A1).

3.5. Efficiency Tests of HDM and STM

The computational time step (Δt) is set to 90 s and is equally divided into 9 sub time steps in the backtracking of the point-wise ELM. The 1-day unsteady flow and sediment transport, under an upstream bankfull discharge (45,000 m^3/s) and a downstream spring tide, is tested to clarify the speedup property of the modeling system. The total runtime of the HDM and the STM is 1550.7 s in sequential runs, and is reduced to 131.1 s in parallel runs ($n_c = 16$) with a speedup of 11.8. The unsteady flow and sediment transport in 1999 are then tested. It takes the modeling system 12.2 h (using 16 cores) to complete the simulation of a 1-year unsteady flow, sediment transport, and riverbed evolution in the Yangtze Estuary.

4. Results

The mechanics of spillover of water and sediment in the Yangtze Estuary are quantitatively studied by simulating typical tidal processes (e.g., a spring tide or a neap tide).

4.1. Simulation Conditions

Similar to former studies on the spillover of saltwater, the spillover of sediment in the Yangtze Estuary is studied using the condition of a spring and a neap tide in dry seasons, when the sediment spillover in the Yangtze Estuary is considered to be most significant.

At the upstream boundary, the river discharge and sediment concentration are set to 19,000 m^3/s and 0.112 kg/m^3, respectively. The flow and sediment fluxes at Datong are then respectively calculated to be 16.41 × 10^8 m^3 and 18.39 × 10^4 tons per day. The seaward boundaries are forced by the tide-level histories of a spring tide and a neap tide, respectively, which leads to two tests of 1-day simulation. Nine cross-sections are arranged to record the histories of the flow rates and the sediment transport rates (see Figure 3). For the sake of convenience, the divisions of North Branch are defined as follows: the upper reach (from the bifurcation of North and South Branches to Station QLG); the middle reach (from Station QLG to SHG); the lower reach (from Station SHG to STG); the tail reach (from Station STG to LXG).

4.2. Horizontal Circulation of Water Flux

The history of the flow rate at cross-sections is integrated over the floodtide and the ebbtide periods to produce the cross-sectional water fluxes (CSWF), as listed in Table 2. According to the simulation results, the reasons for the spillover of water from the North to the South Branches are analyzed in two terms.

Table 2. Cross-sectional water fluxes (*CSWF*) at tide stations (unit: $\times 10^8$ m^3/day).

Region	Cross-Section	Spring Tide		Neap Tide	
		Flood	Ebb	Flood	Ebb
River	JY	−7.72 [1]	24.20	−3.25	19.68
	XLJ	−28.26	44.57	−15.03	31.39
North Branch	QLG	−2.48	1.88	−1.63	1.16
	SHG	−5.73	5.14	−3.22	2.76
	STG	−11.06	10.48	−6.26	5.80
South Branch	SE	−31.41	48.35	−16.34	33.18
	NM	−38.79	55.64	−18.96	35.82
	North C.	−28.52	36.05	−13.09	21.15
	South C.	−25.32	34.61	−11.36	20.21

[1] Note: In the table, a negative value means the direction of the flux is landward, while a positive value means the direction of the flux is seaward. Arrangements of the cross-sections are shown in Figure 3.

First, the tail reach of the North Branch is trumpet-shaped with a wide mouth, in favor of accommodating a great deal of landward tidal flows during floodtide durations. At the same time, the valid river width of the North Branch decreases from the downstream to the upstream, which is accordingly 5–8 km (tail reach), 3–5 km (lower reach), 1–3 km (middle reach), and 1 km (upper reach). Although the *CSWF* at QLG is only 22.4–26.0% of that at STG during floodtide durations, the huge landward floodtide discharge at the mouth of the North Branch and the fast shrinking river width together determine that strong flow intensity can be kept in all the lower, middle, and upper reaches. The velocities in the upper, middle, and lower reaches of North Branch are, respectively, observed to be as large as 2.4, 3.0, and 2.5 m/s, during a floodtide period. The landward floodtide tidal flow moves along the North Branch, while the strong flow intensity is maintained. Finally, some pioneer floodtide flows continue to go through the upper reach of North Branch and arrive at the bifurcation, forming the spillover of water. After a short spillover time, the transition between the floodtide and the ebbtide comes, and the spillover of water is ended.

Second, the upper reach of the North Branch is narrow and almost orthogonal to the South Branch (see Figure 3), which prevents upstream inflows from entering during ebbtide durations. As a result, in upper reach of the North Branch, the seaward ebbtide *CSWF* is smaller than the landward floodtide *CSWF*. At the same time, in the upper reach of the North Branch, the flow intensity during ebbtide durations (maximum velocity, 1.5 m/s) is sharply decreased relative to that during floodtide durations (maximum velocity, 2.4 m/s). The *CSWF* difference between the floodtide and the ebbtide durations at QLG of the North Branch is 0.6–0.47×10^8 m^3/day, accounting for 24.2–28.8% of the landward floodtide *CSWF*. The *CSWF* difference of the North Branch runs downstream along South Branch during ebbtide durations, and a horizontal anticlockwise circulation of water flux is formed.

4.3. Sediment Spillover from North to South Branches

The simulated history of the sediment transport rate at cross-sections is integrated over the floodtide and the ebbtide periods to produce the cross-sectional sediment fluxes (*CSSF*), as listed in Table 3. According to the simulation results, sediment transport of the North Branch, related closely to its hydrodynamics, is analyzed to clarify the mechanics of the sediment spillover from the North to the South Branches.

First, the source of the sediment, which spills over from the North to the South Branches, is recognized. The *CSSF* results show that there exists a critical position of zero sediment flux (ZSF) in the lower reach of North Branch, where the seaward ebbtide *CSSF* just counteracts the landward floodtide *CSSF* in a 1-day runoff-tide process. The ZSF critical position locates about 4 km upstream of STG. Riverbeds in the middle and lower reaches upstream of the ZSF critical position in the North Branch experiences erosions during floodtide durations, corresponding to strong flow intensities there. Sediment concentration of the landward tidal flow is essentially increased during its journey through the erosion reaches of the North Branch. This results in high sediment concentrations of 6–8 kg/m^3 in the reach between QLG and SHG of during floodtide duration in field data. The landward floodtide high-concentration flow, going through cross-section QLG, provides sediment input for the upper reach of North Branch, some of which spillovers from the North to the South Branches.

Table 3. Cross-sectional sediment fluxes (*CSSF*) at tide stations (unit: $\times 10^4$ t/day).

Region	Cross-Section	Spring Tide		Neap Tide	
		Flood	Ebb	Flood	Ebb
River	JY	−10.62 [1]	33.92	−3.31	20.60
	XLJ	−55.76	81.11	−15.28	30.76
North Branch	QLG	−116.73	72.88	−32.28	21.02
	SHG	−244.80	204.47	−56.09	50.97
	STG	−190.93	198.84	−42.65	46.96
South Branch	SE	−85.76	142.00	−19.33	42.69
	NM	−157.33	218.09	−31.61	57.77
	North C.	−130.29	164.43	−20.87	36.27
	South C.	−82.05	109.83	−13.83	25.29

[1] Note: In the table, a negative value means the direction of the flux is landward, while a positive value means the direction of the flux is seaward. Arrangements of the cross-sections are shown in Figure 3.

Second, the kinetic energy of flow, used to advance the spillover of sediment in the Yangtze Estuary, is analyzed. During a floodtide period, the landward flow still maintains considerate intensity (flow velocity) in the upper reach of the North Branch, and at the same time, provides enough kinetic energy for carrying and transporting sediment. The landward floodtide sediment-carrying flow goes through the upper reach of the North Branch and towards the bifurcation. In the journey of the landward flow, partial sediment in the flow deposits on the riverbed along the upper reach of the North Branch, due to the gradually reduced flow intensity. The left part of the sediment in the landward flow arrives at the bifurcation and then spills over to the South Branch.

The process of the sediment spillover in the Yangtze Estuary experiences the following stages. After the floodtide period begins, it takes about 5 h to form the high-concentration floodtide flows in the middle North Branch. The high-concentration floodtide flow arrives at QLG at about 6 h after the floodtide, and begins to spill over to the South Branch at about 7 h. After that, the sediment spillover lasts about 3 h. Then, the transition between the flood and the ebbtides comes, and the sediment spillover gradually disappears.

Third, in the upper reach of the North Branch, the *CSWF* and the flow intensity during ebbtide durations are both sharply reduced relative to those during floodtide durations. The seaward ebbtide *CSSF* is also much smaller than the landward floodtide *CSSF* in the upper reach of the North Branch. The *CSSF* difference between the floodtide and the ebbtide durations at Station QLG is 43.85–11.26 $\times 10^4$ t/day, accounting for 37.5–34.9% of the landward floodtide *CSSF*. The *CSSF* difference of the North Branch is caused by the sediment which spills over from the North to the South Branches. The sediment, arising from the spillover, runs downstream toward the coast along with the ebbtide flow of the South Branch, and a horizontal anticlockwise circulation of sediment flux is formed.

Mechanics of sediment spillover in the Yangtze Estuary can be summarized as a successive process comprising the source, transport, and drainage of the sediment of the spillover.

4.4. Balances of Water and Sediment Fluxes

Using the simulation results (see Video S1 for details), the spatial distributions of water and sediment fluxes in the Yangtze Estuary are sketched, as shown in Figure 11. The horizontal circulations of the water and the sediment fluxes are quantitatively analyzed as follows.

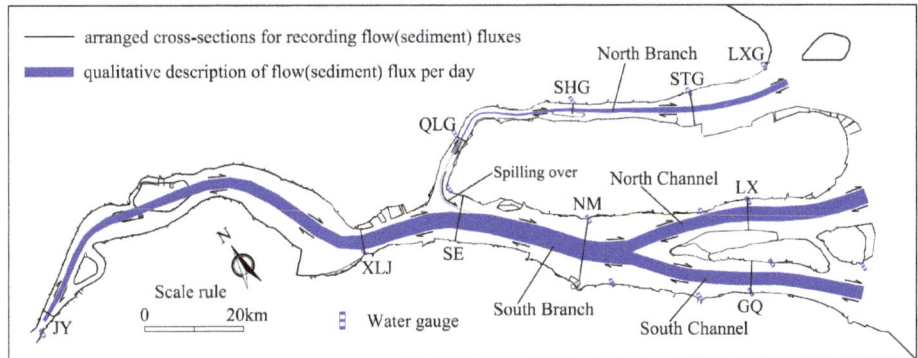

Figure 11. Sketch of the spatial distributions of water and sediment fluxes in Yangtze Estuary.

For a spring tide, the ebbtide *CSWF* at the entrance cross-section of the South Branch (SE) comprises three parts. Water flux, which intrudes upstream of cross-section SE from the South Branch during the floodtide duration, returns during the ebbtide duration and contributes to the first part (31.41 × 10^8 m^3/day). Inflow runoff from Datong (16.31 × 10^8 m^3/day) contributes to the second part. The water spillover from the North Branch (0.6 × 10^8 m^3/day) contributes to the third part, accounting for 1.24% of the ebbtide *CSWF* at cross-section SE. The ebbtide *CSSF* at the entrance cross-section of the South Branch (SE) also comprises three parts. Sediment flux, which intrudes upstream of cross-section SE from the South Branch during the floodtide duration, returns during the ebbtide duration, and contributes to the first part (85.76 × 10^4 t/day). Sediment input at Datong is 18.39 × 10^4 t/day and it evolves to 25.35 × 10^4 t/day at cross-section XLJ after a long-distance adjustment of erosion and deposition, which contributes to the second part. The sediment spillover from North Branch (30.89 × 10^4 t/day) contributes to the third part, accounting for 21.75% of the ebbtide *CSSF* at cross-section SE.

For a neap tide, the water spillover from the North Branch reduces to 0.46 × 10^8 m^3/day, accounting for 1.39% of the *CSWF* at cross-section SE during the ebbtide duration. At the same time, the sediment spillover from the North Branch reduces to 7.88 × 10^4 t/day, accounting for 18.46% of the *CSSF* at cross-section SE during the ebbtide duration.

4.5. Analysis of Spillover on Morphological Dynamics

The riverbed evolution around the bifurcation of the North and the South Branches, which closely relates to the spillover of water and sediment, is qualitatively analyzed, based on the simulation results and the aforementioned spillover mechanics.

When the landward floodtide high-concentration flow goes through the entrance reach of the North Branch, some of the sediment deposits on the riverbed on its landward journey through the upper reach of North Branch and the other part spills over to the South Branch. Overall, for the North Branch, the deposition at the entrance reach will facilitate the shrinkage of its upper reach and further prevent upstream inflows from entering during the ebbtide duration. This conclusion is consistent with field observations and former studies [5,30,35–38].

The entrance reach from the bifurcation to the QLG in the North Branch has a compound floodplain-channel cross-section (see Figure 3), where riverbed evolution may have the following properties. On the one hand, most of the floodtide flow goes through the main channel, and considerate flow intensity is kept there. As a result, it is not easy for the sediment to deposit in the main channel. On the other hand, according to the simulated velocity field of the floodtide flow, the flow intensity of the floodplain is much weaker than that of the main channel, which implies that widespread sediment deposition may happen there.

The morphological dynamics of the North Branch can be summarized as the entrance reach of North Branch will experience successive sediment deposition (the possible sediment deposition mainly happens in the floodplain), leading to shrinkage of the branch.

5. Discussion

5.1. Calculation of Hydrodynamics in Estuaries

The estuary is a transitional region which connects the inland rivers and coastal regions, and is still often regarded as a shallow water system. In existing studies, the nonhydrostatic models and the SWE models are both widely used to simulate estuarine flows.

Relative to SWE models, 3D nonhydrostatic models can include influences of nonhydrostatic pressures which are significant when the ratio of the vertical scale to horizontal scale of motions of flows is not small. Examples are flows over abruptly changing bed topographies, flows with sharp density gradients, and short-wave motions (e.g., waves in coastal and ocean regions). In these cases, the hydrostatic assumption is no longer valid. A short review of certain kinds of 3D nonhydrostatic models can be found in the authors' former studies [9]. Generally, for shallow water systems such as estuary regions, the results simulated by an SWE model are quite similar to those by a 3D nonhydrostatic model. Moreover, a 3D nonhydrostatic model (e.g., 10 layers are used in vertical direction) is at least tens of times slower than a 2D SWE model. It may take more than a month to complete a high-resolution simulation of the 2011–2013 process of the flow, sediment transport, and riverbed evolution in the Yangtze Estuary using the current computing technology used in this paper. Without resorting to simplified methods (e.g., local models, morphological scale factors), high-resolution simulations of long-term processes of flow and sediment transport in the entire Yangtze Estuary using a 3D nonhydrostatic model have not yet been reported.

The SWE models, applied to simulations of estuarine flows, include the 2D SWE models [8,10,13, 18,19,39–41] and the 3D SWE model (e.g., [12,23,24,42–45]). The two kinds of SWE models both use the hydrostatic assumption. On the one hand, high-resolution simulations of short-term processes of tides (e.g., [39,41]), salinity transport (e.g., [8,40–44]), pollutant transport (e.g., [45]) and sediment concentration fields at selected times (e.g., [46]) in the Yangtze Estuary have been gradually enabled due to continuous improvements in computers in the past two decades. On the other hand, the huge computation cost, brought about by simulations of long-term fluvial processes in the Yangtze Estuary using high-resolution grids and small time steps, still challenges most existing 2D/3D numerical codes. In real applications, most of the simulations of hydrodynamics of the Yangtze Estuary take two steps. First, the seaward open boundaries are forced by the time series of tidal levels which are predicted by a GTM such as in [29]. Second, the hydrodynamics of the estuary are simulated by 2D or 3D SWE models. As a result, simulations of the ocean waves, which may be characterized by strong nonhydrostatic pressures and beyond the estuary regions, are in essence not needed. Hence, the application of time-consuming nonhydrostatic 3D models can be totally avoided.

Following the existing studies using SWE models, we adopted a 2D SWE model to perform the simulation of the flow and sediment transport in the Yangtze Estuary in this paper.

5.2. Calculation of Sediment Transport in Estuaries

SWE models for the free-surface flow and sediment transport may be divided into three kinds, which are the Level-1 (the so-called "coupled" model), Level-2 (decoupled model with timely riverbed update, which is used in this paper), and Level-3 (decoupled model using a morphological scale factor) models. These models are compared as follows.

(1) The Level-1 model

The governing equations of the HDM in a Level-1 model can be regarded as an extended version of the SWEs by inserting additional terms, mainly including the density gradient terms and the terms related to the $\partial z_b/\partial t$ (z_b is riverbed elevation). However, the effects of these additional terms are still open issues. Some researchers [47,48] included both of the two kinds of additional terms in their models. Wu [49] pointed out that the effect of the $\partial z_b/\partial t$ term, added into the continuity equation, is dominant relative to the effect of other additional terms. This point is supported in Cao et al. [50], where only the enhanced continuity equation is used together with the momentum equations from the original SWEs. Generally, the Level-1 model is mainly used when the flow, sediment transport, and morphological evolution are strongly coupled to each other (the rate of bed deformation being considerable compared to that of flow evolution), such as the dam-break flows on a moveable riverbed.

(2) The Level-3 model

Notable evolutions of estuarine morphology generally take days, months, or even years, which is much slower than the variations of flow and sediment concentration fields. Impacts of short-term morphology evolutions of riverbeds on tidal currents and sediment transport are also minor. Using these facts, an accelerated calculation of bed deformations could be incorporated in sediment models through multiplying the flux of sediment exchange (between the flow and the riverbed) by a morphological scale factor [10,13,14]. This kind of model is called the Level-3 model.

For a Level-3 model, upstream boundary conditions (e.g., river discharges and sediment concentrations) of a given time interval are set with the average data in this time interval (often a month). Monthly averaged data is used to set the upstream boundary conditions, while water levels of two full-period neap-spring tides are imposed at seaward boundaries. As a result, for each month, only the process of two full neap-spring tides is simulated, and the bed deformation is scaled by a morphological scale factor. Obviously, a Level-3 model using a morphological scale factor does not simulate the real process of the flow, sediment transport, and bed evolution in the estuary.

(3) The Level-2 model

On the one hand, in an estuary, the rate of bed deformation is generally much slower than that of flow evolution, so a Level-1 model is not necessary. On the other hand, the Level-3 model does not simulate a real process of flow-sediment-riverbed evolution. In this study, the real hydrological and tidal processes are simulated. At each time step of a simulation, the calculation of hydrodynamics is done first, and the sediment transport is then solved, followed by a timely riverbed update. This kind of model is called the Level-2 model. Obviously, it is simpler than the Level-1 model and is expected to achieve higher accuracy than the widely used Level-3 model.

5.3. Differences between the Spillover of Saltwater and Sediment

A few quantitative studies on the spillover of saltwater from the North to the South Branches have been reported. Gu et al. [51] found that the spillover of saltwater might occur when the upstream runoff was less than 30,000 m^3/s and the tidal range at Station QLG was greater than 2 m, and became remarkable when the upstream runoff was less than 20,000 m^3/s and the tidal range at Station QLG was greater than 2.5 m. The mechanics and quantitative studies on the spillover of saltwater from the North to the South Branches can be found in [5]. These research results provide references for our study on the spillover of sediment-carrying flow.

It must be pointed that the spillover of sediment in the Yangtze Estuary is quite different from that of saltwater. First, the source for the saltwater spillover is simply from seas, which is uniform at offshore boundaries. As stated in this study, the source for the sediment spillover is produced by the erosion of local riverbed mainly in the middle and upper reaches of the North Branch. Second, salinity can be regarded as a solute whose transport is assumed to fully follow the motion of flows. However, the transport of sediment is quite sensitive to flow intensities. Under weak flow intensity, the heavier particles of sediment will deposit on the riverbed. The flow intensity will determine if and when spillover occurs and its extent. Moreover, the intensity of the sediment spillover is also closely related to the constituents of bed materials. Studies on the sediment spillover are more challenging. This may be one reason that quantitative studies on the sediment spillover in the Yangtze Estuary have not been reported.

According to the aforementioned analysis, a qualified simulation of flow and sediment transport in the Yangtze Estuary (which can reproduce detailed fields of tidal flows and sediment concentration) generally requires a grid resolution higher than that used in the simulation of saltwater transport. High grid resolution is achieved with as few cells as possible by using a channel-refined unstructured grid in this study. Moreover, the semi-implicit method, the ELM, and the FVELM were combined to achieve solve the efficiency problems of the model.

6. Conclusions

To quantitatively clarify the problem of sediment spillover in Yangtze Estuary, a 2D numerical model using a high-resolution channel-refined unstructured grid (200,000 cells) was developed for the entire Yangtze Estuary from Datong to river mouths (620 km) and part of the East Sea. The developed model achieves a good description of the river-coast-ocean coupling, irregular boundaries, and local river regimes in the Yangtze Estuary. The model parameters are calibrated using field data, for which the sensitivity studies are done. In validation tests, the simulated histories of the tidal level, depth-averaged velocity, and sediment concentration agree well with the field data. In efficiency tests, it takes the model 12.2 h (using 16 cores) to complete a simulation of a 1-year unsteady flow, sediment transport, and riverbed evolution in the Yangtze Estuary.

The sediment spillover in the Yangtze Estuary was studied using the conditions of a spring and neap tide in dry seasons. The fluxes of water and sediment at cross-sections are respectively calculated using the simulated histories of flow rates and sediment transport rates. For a representative cross-section in the upper reach of the North Branch (QLG), the difference of the cross-sectional water flux ($CSWF$) between the floodtide and the ebbtide durations is 0.6–0.47 × 10^8 m^3/day, accounting for 24.2–28.8% of the landward floodtide $CSWF$. The difference of the cross-sectional sediment flux ($CSSF$) between the floodtide and the ebbtide durations is 43.85–11.26 × 10^4 t/day, accounting for 37.5–34.9% of the landward floodtide $CSSF$.

The mechanics of sediment spillover in the Yangtze Estuary are summarized as a successive process comprising the source, transport, and drainage of the sediment of the spillover.

Supplementary Materials: The following are available online at http://www.mdpi.com/2077-1312/7/11/390/s1, Figure S1: Channel-refined computational grid for numerical model of Yangtze Estuary. Video S1: Process of the spillover of sediment from the North to the South Branches during a full spring tide in Yangtze Estuary.

Author Contributions: Conceptualization: D.H. and Z.J.; methodology: D.H. and Z.J.; software: D.H. and M.W.; validation: D.H., M.W. and Z.J.; formal analysis: D.H., M.W. and Z.J.; investigation: D.H. and Z.J.; resources: S.Y. and Z.J.; data curation: S.Y. and D.H.; writing—original draft preparation: D.H. and Z.J.; writing—review and editing: M.W. and D.H.; visualization: M.W.; supervision: S.Y. and Z.J.; project administration: S.Y. and Z.J.; funding acquisition: D.H., S.Y. and Z.J.

Funding: Financial support from Science and Technology Program of Guizhou Province, China (Grant No. 2017-3005-4), the Fundamental Research Funds for the Central Universities (2017KFYXJJ197), China's National Natural Science Foundation (51339001, 51779015 and 51479009) are acknowledged.

Conflicts of Interest: The authors declare no conflict of interest.

References

1. He, S.L.; Sun, J.M. Characteristics of suspended sediment transport in the turbidity maximum of the Changjiang river estuary. *Oceanol. Limnol. Sin.* **1996**, *27*, 60–66. (In Chinese)
2. Li, J.F.; Shi, W.R.; Shen, H.T. Sediment properties and transportation in the turbidity maximum in Changjiang estuary. *Geogr. Res.* **1994**, *13*, 51–59. (In Chinese)
3. Shen, J.; Shen, H.T.; Pan, D.A.; Xiao, C.Y. Analysis of transport mechanism of water and suspended sediment in the turbidity maximum of the Changjiang estuary. *Acta Geogr. Sin.* **1995**, *50*, 412–420. (In Chinese)

4. Shi, Z.; Chen, M.W. Fine sediment transport in turbidity maximum at the north passage of the Changjiang Estuary. *J. Sediment Res.* **2000**, *1*, 28–39. (In Chinese)
5. Wu, H.; Zhu, J.R.; Chen, B.R.; Chen, Y.Z. Quantitative relationship of runoff and tide to saltwater spilling over from the North Branch in the Changjiang Estuary, A numerical study. *Estuar. Coast. Shelf Sci.* **2006**, *69*, 125–132. [CrossRef]
6. Chen, W.; Li, J.F.; Li, Z.H.; Li, Z.H.; Dai, Z.J.; Yan, H.; Xu, M.; Zhao, J.K. The suspended sediment transportation and its mechanism in strong tidal reaches of the North Branch of the Changjiang Estuary. *Acta Oceanol. Sin.* **2012**, *34*, 84–91. (In Chinese)
7. Chen, C.S.; Xue, P.F.; Ding, P.X.; Beardsley, R.C.; Xu, Q.C.; Mao, X.M.; Gao, G.P.; Qi, J.H.; Li, C.Y.; Lin, H.C.; et al. Physical mechanisms for the offshore detachment of the Changjiang Diluted Water in the East China Sea. *J. Geophys. Res.* **2008**, *113*. [CrossRef]
8. Xue, P.F.; Chen, C.S.; Ding, P.X.; Beardsley, R.C.; Lin, H.C.; Ge, J.Z.; Kong, Y.Z. Saltwater intrusion into the Changjiang River, A model-guided mechanism study. *J. Geophys. Res.* **2009**, *114*. [CrossRef]
9. Hu, D.C.; Wang, G.Q.; Zhang, H.W.; Zhong, D.Y. A semi-implicit three-dimensional numerical model for non-hydrostatic pressure free-surface flows on an unstructured, sigma grid. *Int. J. Sediment Res.* **2013**, *28*, 77–89. [CrossRef]
10. Hu, K.L.; Ding, P.X.; Wang, Z.B.; Yang, S.L. A 2D/3D hydrodynamic and sediment transport model for the Yangtze Estuary, China. *J. Mar. Syst.* **2009**, *77*, 114–136. [CrossRef]
11. Shi, Z.; Zhou, H.Q.; Liu, H.; Zhang, Y.C. Two-dimensional horizontal modeling of fine-sediment transport at the South Channel–North Passage of the partially mixed Changjiang River Estuary, China. *Environ. Earth Sci.* **2010**, *61*, 1691–1702. [CrossRef]
12. Zuo, S.H.; Zhang, N.C.; Li, B.; Zhang, Z.; Zhu, Z.X. Numerical simulation of tidal current and erosion and sedimentation in the Yangshan deep-water harbor of Shanghai. *Int. J. Sediment Res.* **2009**, *24*, 287–298. [CrossRef]
13. Kuang, C.P.; Liu, X.; Gu, J.; Guo, Y.K.; Huang, S.C.; Liu, S.G.; Yu, W.W.; Huang, J.; Sun, B. Numerical prediction of medium-term tidal flat evolution in the Yangtze Estuary, impacts of the Three Gorges project. *Cont. Shelf Res.* **2013**, *52*, 12–26. [CrossRef]
14. WL|Delft Hydraulics. *Delft3D-FLOW User Manual*; Version 3.13; WL|Delft Hydraulics: Delft, The Netherlands, 2006.
15. Wang, D.Z. Transport of Nonuniform Bedload in the Changjiang Estuary and Its Numerical Simulation. Master's Thesis, Zhejiang University, Zhejiang, China, 2002. (In Chinese).
16. Han, Q.W.; He, M.M. *The Statistics Theory of Sediment Transport*; Chinese Science Press: Beijing, China, 1984. (In Chinese)
17. Cheng, C.; Huang, H.M.; Liu, C.Y.; Jiang, W.M. Challenges to the representation of suspended sediment transfer using a depth-averaged flux. *Earth Surf. Proc. Land.* **2016**, *41*, 1337–1357. [CrossRef]
18. Dou, X.P.; Li, T.L.; Dou, G.R. Numerical model of total sediment transport in the Yangtze Estuary. *China Ocean Eng.* **1999**, *13*, 277–286.
19. Wan, Y.Y.; Roelvink, D.; Li, W.H.; Qi, D.M.; Gu, F.F. Observation and modeling of the storm-induced fluid mud dynamics in a muddy-estuarine navigational channel. *Geomorphology* **2014**, *217*, 23–36. [CrossRef]
20. Xie, J.; Yan, Y.X. Promoting siltation effects and impacts of Hengsha East. *J. Hydrodyn.* **2011**, *23*, 649–659. [CrossRef]
21. Zhang, R.J.; Xie, J.H. *River Sediment Transport*; Press of Chinese Hydraulic and Electric Engineering: Beijing, China, 1989. (In Chinese)
22. Wei, Z.L.; Zhao, L.K.; Fu, X.P. Research on mathematical model for sediment in Yellow River. *J. Wuhan Univ. Hydr. Electr. Eng.* **1997**, *30*, 21–25. (In Chinese)
23. Zhang, Y.L.; Baptista, A.M.; Myers, E.P. A cross-scale model for 3D baroclinic circulation in estuary-plume-shelf systems, I. Formulation and skill assessment. *Cont. Shelf Res.* **2004**, *24*, 2187–2214. [CrossRef]
24. Casulli, V.; Walters, R.A. An unstructured grid, three-dimensional model based on the shallow water equations. *Int. J. Numer. Meth. Fluids* **2000**, *32*, 331–348. [CrossRef]
25. Hu, D.C.; Zhong, D.Y.; Zhang, H.W.; Wang, G.Q. Prediction–correction method for parallelizing implicit 2D hydrodynamic models I scheme. *J. Hydraul. Eng.* **2015**, *141*, 04015014. [CrossRef]
26. Hu, D.C.; Zhong, D.Y.; Zhu, Y.H.; Wang, G.Q. Prediction–correction method for parallelizing implicit 2D hydrodynamic models II application. *J. Hydraul. Eng.* **2015**, *141*, 06015008. [CrossRef]

27. Dimou, K. 3-D Hybrid Eulerian–Lagrangian/Particle Tracking Model for Simulating Mass Transport in Coastal Water Bodies. Ph.D. Thesis, Massachusetts Institute of Technology, Cambridge, MA, USA, 1992.
28. Hu, D.C.; Zhu, Y.H.; Zhong, D.Y.; Qin, H. Two-dimensional finite-volume Eulerian-Lagrangian method on unstructured grid for solving advective transport of passive scalars in free-surface flows. *J. Hydraul. Eng.* **2017**, *143*, 04017051. [CrossRef]
29. Cheng, Y.C.; Andersen, O.B.; Knudsen, P. Integrating non-tidal sea level data from altimetry and tide gauges for coastal sea level prediction. *Adv. Space Res.* **2012**, *50*, 1099–1106. [CrossRef]
30. Wu, S.H.; Cheng, H.Q.; Xu, Y.J.; Li, J.F.; Zheng, S.W.; Xu, W. Riverbed micromorphology of the Yangtze River Estuary, China. *Water* **2016**, *8*, 190. [CrossRef]
31. Cao, Z.Y. A Two-Dimensional Non-Uniform Sediment Numerical Model for the Yangtze Estuary. Ph.D. Thesis, East China Normal University, Shanghai, China, 2003. (In Chinese).
32. Shi, Y.B.; Lu, H.Y.; Yang, Y.P.; Cao, Y. Prediction of erosion depth under the action of the exceptional flood in the river reach of a tunnel across the Qiantang estuary. *Adv. Water Sci.* **2008**, *19*, 685–692. (In Chinese)
33. Baptista, A.M. Solution of Advection-Dominated Transport by Eulerian–Lagrangian Methods Using the Backwards Method of Characteristics. Ph.D. Thesis, Massachusetts Institute of Technology, Cambridge, MA, USA, 1987.
34. Hu, D.C.; Zhang, H.W.; Zhong, D.Y. Properties of the Eulerian-Lagrangian method using linear interpolators in a three dimensional shallow water model using z-level coordinates. *Int. J. Comput. Fluid Dyn.* **2009**, *23*, 271–284. [CrossRef]
35. Li, Z.H.; Li, M.Z.; Dai, Z.J.; Zhao, F.F.; Li, J.F. Intratidal and neap-spring variations of suspended sediment concentrations and sediment transport processes in the North Branch of the Changjiang Estuary. *Acta Oceanol. Sin.* **2015**, *34*, 137–147. [CrossRef]
36. Liu, H.; He, Q.; Wang, Z.B.; Weltje, G.J.; Zhang, J. Dynamics and spatial variability of near-bottom sediment exchange in the Yangtze Estuary, China. *Estuar. Coast. Shelf Sci.* **2010**, *86*, 322–330. [CrossRef]
37. Shi, Z.; Zhang, S.Y.; Hamilton, L.J. Bottom fine sediment boundary layer and transport processes at the mouth of the Changjiang Estuary, China. *J. Hydrol.* **2006**, *327*, 276–288. [CrossRef]
38. Yang, S.L.; Belkinb, I.M.; Belkinac, A.I.; Zhao, Q.Y.; Zhu, J.; Ding, P.X. Delta response to decline in sediment supply from the Yangtze River: Evidence of the recent four decades and expectations for the next half-century. *Estuar. Coast. Shelf Sci.* **2003**, *57*, 689–699. [CrossRef]
39. Tan, Y.; Yang, F.; Xie, D.H. The change of tidal characteristics under the influence of human activities in the Yangtze Estuary. *J. Coast. Res.* **2016**, *75*, 163–167. [CrossRef]
40. Wu, D.; Shao, Y.; Pan, J. Study on activities and concentration of saline group in the South Branch in Yangtze River Estuary. *Procedia Eng.* **2015**, *116*, 1085–1094.
41. Lu, S.; Tong, C.; Lee, D.Y.; Zheng, J.; Shen, J.; Zhang, W.; Yan, Y. Propagation of tidal waves up in Yangtze Estuary during the dry season. *J. Geophys. Res. Oceans* **2015**, *120*, 6445–6473. [CrossRef]
42. Ge, J.Z.; Ding, P.X.; Chen, C.S. Low-salinity plume detachment under non-uniform summer wind off the Changjiang Estuary. *Estuar. Coast. Shelf Sci.* **2015**, *156*, 61–70. [CrossRef]
43. Hou, C.C.; Zhu, J.R. The response time of saltwater intrusion in the Changjiang River to the change of river discharge in dry season. *Acta Oceanol. Sin.* **2013**, *35*, 29–35. (In Chinese)
44. An, Q.; Wu, Y.Q.; Taylor, S.; Zhao, B. Influence of the Three Gorges Project on saltwater intrusion in the Yangtze River Estuary. *Environ. Geol.* **2009**, *56*, 1679–1686. [CrossRef]
45. Zhang, J.X.; Liu, H. Numerical investigation of pollutant transport by tidal flow in the Yangtze Estuary. In *Trends in Engineering Mechanics Special Publication*; Huang, W., Wang, K., Chen, Q., Eds.; American Society of Civil Engineers: Los Angeles, CA, USA, 2010; pp. 99–110.
46. Kuang, C.P.; Chen, W.; Gu, J.; He, L.L. Comprehensive analysis on the sediment siltation in the upper reach of the deepwater navigation channel in the Yangtze Estuary. *J. Hydrodyn.* **2014**, *26*, 299–308. [CrossRef]
47. Zhang, S.; Duan, J.; Strelkoff, T. Grain-scale nonequilibrium sediment-transport model for unsteady flow. *J. Hydraul. Eng.* **2012**, *139*, 22–36. [CrossRef]
48. Xia, J.Q.; Lin, B.L.; Falconer, R.A.; Wang, G.Q. Modelling dam-break flows over mobile beds using a 2D coupled approach. *Adv. Water Res.* **2010**, *33*, 171–183. [CrossRef]
49. Wu, W.M. Earthen embankment breaching. *J. Hydraul. Eng.* **2011**, *137*, 1549–1564.

50. Cao, Z.; Pender, G.; Wallis, S.; Carling, P. Computational dam-break hydraulics over erodible sediment bed. *J. Hydraul. Eng.* **2004**, *130*, 689–703. [CrossRef]
51. Gu, Y.; Wu, S.; Yue, Q. Impact of intruded saline water via North Branch of the Yangtze River on water source areas in the estuary area. *Yangtze River* **2003**, *34*, 1–16. (In Chinese)

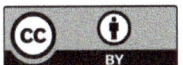

© 2019 by the authors. Licensee MDPI, Basel, Switzerland. This article is an open access article distributed under the terms and conditions of the Creative Commons Attribution (CC BY) license (http://creativecommons.org/licenses/by/4.0/).

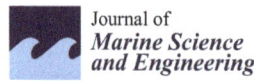

Article

Critical Processes of Trace Metals Mobility in Transitional Waters: Implications from the Remote, Antinioti Lagoon, Corfu Island, Greece

Fotini Botsou [1,*], Aristomenis P. Karageorgis [2], Vasiliki Paraskevopoulou [1], Manos Dassenakis [1] and Michael Scoullos [1]

1. Laboratory of Environmental Chemistry, Department of Chemistry, National and Kapodistrian University of Athens, 15784 Athens, Greece
2. Institute of Oceanography, Hellenic Centre for Marine Research, 19013 Anavyssos, Greece
* Correspondence: fbotsou@chem.uoa.gr; Tel.: +30-210-727-4951

Received: 6 August 2019; Accepted: 2 September 2019; Published: 4 September 2019

Abstract: The Antinioti Lagoon is a karstified, rather pristine, and shallow coastal lagoon located in the northern part of Corfu Island in NW Greece. The present study examines the levels of metals (Al, Fe, Mn, Cd, Cu, Pb, and Zn) in the dissolved and particulate phase, as well as in surface and core sediments, and identifies the critical processes that define their behavior. The major transport pathway of dissolved Mn, Cd, and Pb, and particulate Mn, Cd, and Zn into the lagoon is through freshwater springs, whereas surface runoff dominates the transport of particulate Al, Fe, and Cu. Interestingly, large particles (>8 μm) contain higher amounts of Al, Fe and Mn than the finer ones (<8 μm), due to flocculation of oxyhydroxides that, eventually, scavenge other metals, as well. Cadmium and Zn bound to the large particles were found to be less prone to desorption than the smaller ones and were effectively captured within the lagoon. In the sediments, diagenetic processes are responsible for post-depositional changes in the forms of metals (particularly Fe, Mn and Cd). Enrichment factors (EFs) based on local background showed that sediments are enriched in restricted areas in Cd and Pb by maximum factors 4.8 and 10, respectively. These metals were predominantly found in potentially labile forms. Thus, any interventions introducing changes in the physico-chemical conditions may result in the release of metals, with negative implications on the lagoon's ecological quality.

Keywords: coastal lagoon; dissolved and particulate metals; sediments; labile forms; enrichment factor; early diagenetic process; groundwater discharges

1. Introduction

Trace metals enter coastal lagoons through several pathways, such as atmospheric depositions [1], industrial and urban discharges [2,3], agricultural run-off [4,5], riverine inputs [6], groundwater discharges [7], as well as benthic fluxes [8,9]. Upon reaching the lagoons, trace metals, under variable physicochemical gradients, participate in a series of complex physical, geochemical, and biological processes that greatly affect the distribution of trace metals over the particulate and dissolved phases, as well as the composition of the deposited sediment, and eventually, the fluxes of metals that reach the adjacent sea. These critical biogeochemical processes include complexation reactions of trace metals with dissolved organic and inorganic ligands, adsorption/desorption reactions onto inorganic and organic suspended particles, flocculation and coagulation of colloidal and particulate species, and remobilization from sediments. All these processes vary with pH, ionic strength, the amount and the composition of suspended particles, as well as with redox conditions [10,11].

The limited water exchange with the open sea and the dominant low energy regime from tides, waves and currents, favors the long residence time of water and suspended particulate matter at the fresh − saline water interface, which in turn, kinetically enables the chemical reactions between the dissolved and particulate phase to take place [12]. Furthermore, the prevailing low energy hydrological regime, favors the accumulation of major and trace elements in sediments [2,13] as well as the accumulation of high amounts of organic matter of autochthonous and allochthonous origin [14,15]. Oxidation of organic matter directly influences the redox potential of the sediment pore water [15]. Once oxygen is consumed, the oxidation of organic matter proceeds via other oxidants following the theoretical sequence: $O_2 > NO_3/MnO_2 > Fe(OH)_3 > SO_4^{2-}$ [16,17]. Diagenetic processes may have a profound, direct or indirect, effect on the mobility, thus the bioavailability of trace elements [1,18,19]. The remobilization of trace metals occurs principally when Fe and Mn oxyhydroxides are reduced, but such remobilization can be partially or totally prevented in the presence of sulfide, which reacts to form metal sulfide complexes whose solubility controls the fraction of metals dissolved in solution [17,20]. Furthermore, a number of other natural or anthropogenic disturbances, such as re-suspension of sediments due to storms and waves, eutrophication events, and dredging of sediments, could turn sediments from sinks to a long-term source of contaminants to the water column [4,11], particularly when occurring in shallow settings [21] with potentially hazardous effects for the biota.

The Antinioti Lagoon is a rather remote, non-industrialized, moderately urbanized, shallow coastal system located at the northern part of Corfu (Kerkyra) Island in northwestern Greece. The site is of great ecological significance, and as such, is included in the Natura 2000 network as special area of conservation for Europe and is declared as a Site of Community Importance and Special Protection Area [22]. It is also important for fisheries supplying the local market. Despite its importance, previous studies on the area are rare.

The site is also of scientific interest from the geochemical perspective. In a previous publication it was shown that post-depositional formation of iron sulfide minerals, predominantly pyrite, and incorporation of trace elements into the pyrite phase takes place extensively in deposited sediments, limiting the mobility, and thus the bioavailability of trace metals [23]. In the present study, the distribution of trace metals in three phases, the dissolved, suspended particulate matter, and deposited sediments is examined. The interactions of trace metals between the three phases are investigated in relation to the physicochemical and geochemical parameters. Core sediments are used to estimate the local background levels and reveal temporal trends of accumulation of trace metals due to natural and anthropogenic sources. The main purpose of this study is to identify the critical processes that define trace metals' mobility and fate within the transitional fresh-saline water interface and beyond. In a broader context, the results of the study may contribute to the understanding of the overall behavior of trace metals in similar coastal lagoonal systems, which represent a typical set of transitional ecosystems in the Mediterranean Sea.

2. The Study Area

Antinioti Lagoon (39° 49' N, 19° 52' E) is part of the homonymous wetland consisting of the lagoon itself (40 ha), and marshes and wet meadows (60 ha) that extend to the southeastern part of the lagoon. The lagoon is shallow with depths ranging from 20 cm to 150 cm and communicates with the Ionian Sea through two channels, separated by the Agia Aikaterini Islet (Figure 1).

Besides surface runoff and precipitation, the freshwater inputs included a series of groundwater springs seeping at the bottom of the lake (close to sites A3, A5, A8; Figure 1) with various yields; another spring flows as a surface stream (site A13) discharging at the southeastern part of the lake (hereafter "stream"). These springs are related to the karstified carbonate formations outcropping in the study area [24]. Two major karstic formations are developed: the upper unit of medium permeability represented by Upper Jurassic – Upper Cretaceous Vigla limestones and the underlying highly permeable Jurassic limestones and dolomites of Pantokrator. An impermeable sequence of Jurassic Posidonia schist interposes between the carbonate rocks and influences the penetration of water from the upper carbonate strata to the lower one, as well as the surface water and groundwater flow paths [24,25]. The main solid phase characterization of sediments by powder XRD [23] revealed the abundance of quartz followed by calcite, the presence of common phyllosilicates (clays and micas), traces of dolomite, as well as significant amounts of pyrite. This is in accordance with the previous study by Tserolas et al. [26], describing the geology of the wider area.

The wetland sustains a variety of habitats (marshes and water fringed vegetation) and is important for several species of flora, fauna, in particular avifauna, some of which are endangered. Antinioti Lagoon supports also the local economy, as it is exploited for semi-natural extensive fish farming of mullets, seabreams, and eels. Its catchment area is partly agricultural (mainly olive trees) and partly touristic, with intense seasonality in the tourism flow. The greatest threats to the site and its conservation derive from lack of effective management, combined with: (a) the unauthorized disposal of solid wastes and occasionally of domestic wastewater; (b) the excessive use of fertilizers and pesticides in adjacent cultivated areas (e.g., olive groves); (c) the increase of dwellings and tourist infrastructures; and (d) the lack of awareness of the local community about the importance of the wetland [22].

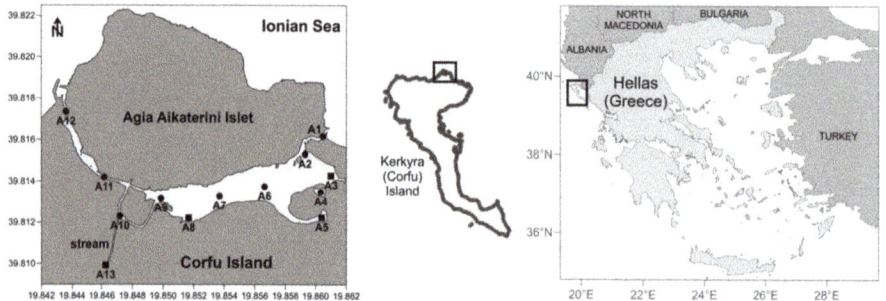

Figure 1. Location of the study area and sampling stations. Rectangles mark groundwater discharges.

3. Materials and Methods

3.1. Sampling

Two sampling campaigns were carried out in May 2006 and May 2007, under calm weather conditions. Water samples were collected during both campaigns, surface sediments were collected during the first campaign, and core sediments were collected during the second one. Two stations at the seawater inlets represent the seaward boundary conditions (A1, A12), one station the freshwater stream (A13), while the rest of the stations represent the conditions in the inner part of the lagoon (A2–A11; Figure 1). *In situ* measurements of temperature, salinity, conductivity, pH, and dissolved oxygen were conducted by YSI 63 and YSI 57 portable instruments throughout the water column.

Water sampling bottles were soaked in 10% HNO_3 for at least 48 h, then thoroughly rinsed with deionized water (18 MΩ·cm) and stored in double polyethylene bags in a laminar flow bench. In the field, the bottles were rinsed twice with ambient water, and then the samples were collected by hand by submersing pre-cleaned polyethylene bottles at up to 20 cm beneath the water surface. During sampling, all necessary precautions were taken to avoid contamination. The samples were transported in two polyethylene bags stored in a portable refrigerator.

Surface sediment samples were collected by an Ekman-Birge grab sampler. A short sediment core was collected from station A8 (Figure 1) with a Plexiglas tube 60 cm-long and 10 cm-wide, attached to a push-tube coring device. The core was sectioned immediately after the collection into 1–2 cm intervals. Sediment samples were stored in pre-cleaned polyethylene vessels and transported in a portable refrigerator.

3.2. Samples Pretreatment

All labware used in the analytical procedures were soaked in 10% HNO_3 for at least 48 h, and then thoroughly rinsed with deionized water. Precautions were taken during all stages in order to avoid contamination.

The water samples were filtered under a clean laminar bench. The filtration was carried out in succession through 8 µm and 0.45 µm Millipore filters in order to separate the dissolved (<0.45 µm) and the particulate phase (>0.45 µm) and determine the suspended particulate matter (SPM) in two grain-size fractions (0.45 µm < diameter (d) < 8 µm and d > 8 µm). The filtrates for the determination of dissolved metals were acidified to pH < 2 by HNO_3 prior to pre-concentration on Chelex-100 (100–200 mesh, BioRad Laboratories) and subsequent elution of trace metals [27].

The filters for particulate metals (0.45 µm < d < 8 µm and d > 8 µm) were dried to constant weight and then digested with concentrated HNO_3 on a hot plate (85 °C approximately) overnight [27].

Sediment samples were freeze-dried in a Labconco apparatus. Then the silt and clay fraction (<63 µm) was separated by means of sieving. This approach has been widely used to reduce the physical variability of metal content due to grain size effects [28–30], although recently its effectiveness has been questioned, particularly if coatings of metal scavengers exist in coarse-grained particles [31]. Total metals contents were determined after complete dissolution of sediments with an acid mixture of HNO_3-$HClO_4$-HF acids [32]. The 0.5 N HCl extractable metals were determined after the method of Agemian and Chau [33].

3.3. Analytical Procedures

Trace metals analysis was performed by means of Flame and Graphite Furnace AAS (Varian SpectrAA-200 and Varian SpectrAA-640 Zeeman) (Varian, Australia), depending on the concentration levels of each determined element. Procedural blanks were run in the same way as samples and were usually below Limits of Detections (LOD), reported in Table 1.

Table 1. Quality assurance data of the methods employed for the determination of metals in the dissolved and particulate phase and total contents in sediments.

Variable	Al	Cd	Cu	Fe	Mn	Pb	Zn
			Dissolved phase				
LOD (µg·L^{-1}) CASS-4:	-	0.0038	0.044	1	0.0085	0.040	0.50
Assigned value	-	0.026 ± 0.003	0.592 ± 0.055	-	2.78 ± 0.19	0.0098 ± 0.0035	0.381 ± 0.057
Measured value	-	0.024 ± 0.002	0.570 ± 0.030	-	2.79 ± 0.12	0.0089 ± 0.0023	0.409 ± 0.030
Recovery% (spikes)	-	106–102–102% at 0.05–0.1–0.2 µg·L^{-1}	99–96–93 at 0.2–1.0–2.0 µg·L^{-1}	73–80 at 5–7.9 µg·L^{-1}	98–98–101 at 0.2–1.0–5.0 µg·L^{-1}	99–93–92 at 0.2–1.0–2.0 µg·L^{-1}	105–101–100 at 1.0–2.0–5.0 µg·L^{-1}
Repeatability% (spikes)	-	6.4% at 0.05 µg·L^{-1} 3.5% at 0.2 µg·L^{-1}	5.4% at 0.2 µg·L^{-1} 1.9% at 2.0 µg·L^{-1}	2.3% at 5 µg·L^{-1} 4.0% at 7.9 µg·L^{-1}	4.8% at 0.2 µg·L^{-1} 2.7% at 5.0 µg·L^{-1}	6.9% at 0.2 µg·L^{-1} 2.8% at 2.0 µg·L^{-1}	5.8% at 1.0 µg·L^{-1} 5.2% at 5.0 µg·L^{-1}
			Particulate phase				
LOD part. metals (µg·L^{-1})	0.62	0.0019	0.022	0.5	0.0042	0.020	0.25
Repeatability%	20% at 50 µg·L^{-1}	12% at 0.0022 µg·L^{-1}	15% at 0.05 µg·L^{-1}	5.5% at 15 µg·L^{-1}	9.6% at 0.13 µg·L^{-1}	5.3% at 0.19 µg·L^{-1}	11% at 0.93 µg·L^{-1}
			Sediments (total digestions)				
LOD (mg·kg^{-1}) PACS-2:	1.7	0.015	0.177	4	0.034	0.16	2
Assigned value	66200 ± 3200	2.11 ± 0.15	310 ± 12	40900 ± 600	440 ± 19	183 ± 8	364 ± 23
Measured value	63000 ± 800	2.2 ± 0.2	300 ± 10	41700 ± 600	440 ± 10	187 ± 8	380 ± 15
Recovery% (PACS-2)	95	104	97	102	99	102	104
Repeatability% (PACS-2)	1.3	6.8	3.3	1.4	2.3	4.3	3.9

The accuracy and repeatability of dissolved metals determinations by the Chelex-100 resin has been tested in the laboratory using spiked seawater samples at three concentration levels, as well as by analyzing the certified reference material (CRM) CASS-4 (from National Research Council of Canada, NRCC) (Table 1). In the case of the sediment samples, the accuracy and repeatability of total sediment digestions was evaluated by analyzing the certified reference materials PACS-2 (NRCC) with satisfactory results (Table 1).

3.4. Statistical Analyses

Statistically significant differences of metal concentrations (dissolved and particulate) among the three sectors of the system, i.e., the inlets, the inner part of the lagoon and the freshwater spring, were explored by independent t-test on log transformed values to correct for departure from normality. The relationships among the considered variables were tested by using non-parametric Spearman coefficient. A probability level below $\varrho < 0.05$ was set as statistically significant. Statistical analyses were carried out using the IBM SPSS software v. 21.0 (IBM corp, Armonk, NY, USA).

4. Results

4.1. Physicochemical Parameters and SPM

Summary statistics of the physicochemical parameters and SPM in the three sectors of the system, the stream, the inner part, and the inlets, is presented in Table 2; the detailed results per each sampling are given in Table A1. Salinity values exhibited significant spatial variation (Table 2) due to mixing of seawater and freshwater. Higher values were found at the inlets (A1 and A12) due to seawater intrusion. During both sampling periods, the western inlet exhibited higher values of salinity than the eastern, signifying that this part of the lagoon is more exposed to sea currents (Table A1). In fact, in the past, considerable amounts of sediments were transferred after strong and persistent northerly winds and sealed the inlet (a feature known as sediment plug), which was artificially re-opened in order to facilitate water circulation and fishing activities. Concerning the inner stations, surface salinity ranged from 8.6 to 17.6. Bottom salinity was higher than in surface layers (data not shown).

At the inlets, pH obtained typical values of seawater (7.9–8.3), whereas the values found at the inner part of lagoon and the stream were 7.5–8.3 and ≤ 7.5, respectively (Table 2).

Table 2. Ranges (min–max) and median values (in parenthesis) of salinity, pH, SPM and dissolved (d.) and particulate (p. in w/w) metals in the three sectors of the Antinioti Lagoon system, during both sampling periods.

Parameter	Stream	Inner Sector	Inlets
salinity	1.70–4.80 (1.75)	8.60–19.4 (13.6)	22.0–37.7 (33.8)
pH	7.26–7.51 (7.38)	7.45–8.30 (7.94)	8.01–8.24 (8.17)
SPM (mg·L^{-1})	1.53–1.95 (1.74)	7.04–14.2 (10.4)	13.4–20.9 (14.6)
d. Fe (µg·L^{-1})	2.61–5.23 (3.92)	0.42–6.32 (1.99)	0.43–6.36 (2.12)
d. Mn (µg·L^{-1})	2.91–15.4 (9.14)	1.32–7.67 (4.31)	1.12–4.36 (1.47)
d. Cd (µg·L^{-1})	0.069–0.164 (0.116)	0.016–0.079 (0.038)	0.018–0.025 (0.019)
d. Cu (µg·L^{-1})	0.16–0.47 (0.32)	0.09–1.53 (0.35)	0.18–0.66 (0.30)
d. Pb (µg·L^{-1})	0.20–0.27 (0.24)	0.02–0.34 (0.08)	0.03–0.06 (0.06)
d. Zn (µg·L^{-1})	3.17–9.94 (6.56)	1.00–15.0 (4.18)	1.20–3.37 (2.35)
p. Al (mg·kg^{-1})	3406–4204 (3805)	4905–90457 (8334)	2432–15629 (7152)
p. Fe (mg·kg^{-1})	6731–12793 (9762)	3496–58612 (6024)	2379–11996 (6279)
p. Mn (mg·kg^{-1})	1667–1945 (1806)	173–1213 (385)	36–258 (109)
p. Cd (mg·kg^{-1})	3.76–5.23 (4.50)	0.63–4.20 (1.84)	0.09–0.78 (0.40)
p. Cu (mg·kg^{-1})	51–101 (76)	10–177 (25.6)	7–22 (19)
p. Pb (mg·kg^{-1})	22.8–36.9 (29.9)	5.91–81.7 (16.2)	7.0–16.5 (10.4)
p. Zn (mg·kg^{-1})	198–1790 (994)	22–423 (193)	12–107 (62)

Suspended Particulate Matter (SPM) concentrations were higher at the inlets than in the inner part of the lagoon (Table 2), due to the turbulent mixing of seawater and fresh/brackish water and the re-suspension of sediments. The lowest concentrations were found at the stream, station A13 (1.5 mg·L^{-1} and 2 mg·L^{-1} in the first and second sampling, respectively). Particles with diameter d > 8 µm accounted for 68 ± 14% (mean ± sd) of total SPM at the inlets, 64 ± 8% of SPM at the inner part of the lagoon, and 38 ± 23% at the stream.

4.2. Trace Metals in Water

4.2.1. Levels and Spatial Variation

The Water Framework Directive 2000/60/EC [34] identified Cd and Pb as priority substances, posing a threat to, or via, the aquatic environment at the EU level. Environmental quality standards (EQS) have been set by its Daughter Directive 2013/39/EU [35] with annual average values for Cd: 0.2 µg·L^{-1} and 1.3 µg·L^{-1} for Pb. The concentrations of dissolved metals in the inner sector and the inlets were well below the EQS (Table 2). However, dissolved Cd in the stream (0.116 µg·L^{-1}) was marginally below the EQS, suggesting that this element is of environmental concern and should be regularly monitored.

The stream, of groundwater origin, was the major source of Cd into the lagoon. This is evidenced by the fact that dissolved, total, i.e., the sum of dissolved and particulate (w/v) shown in Figure 2, as well as particulate (w/w; Table 2) Cd concentrations were significantly higher in the stream than the inner sector. Furthermore, the stream constituted the primary source of dissolved Pb, dissolved and particulate (both in w/w and w/v) Mn, and particulate (w/w) Zn. In contrast, the concentrations of Fe and Pb in the particulate phase (w/v) were significantly higher in the inner sector than the stream, suggesting that other sources (e.g., runoff) rather than the emanating groundwater are responsible for the transport of these elements into the lagoon.

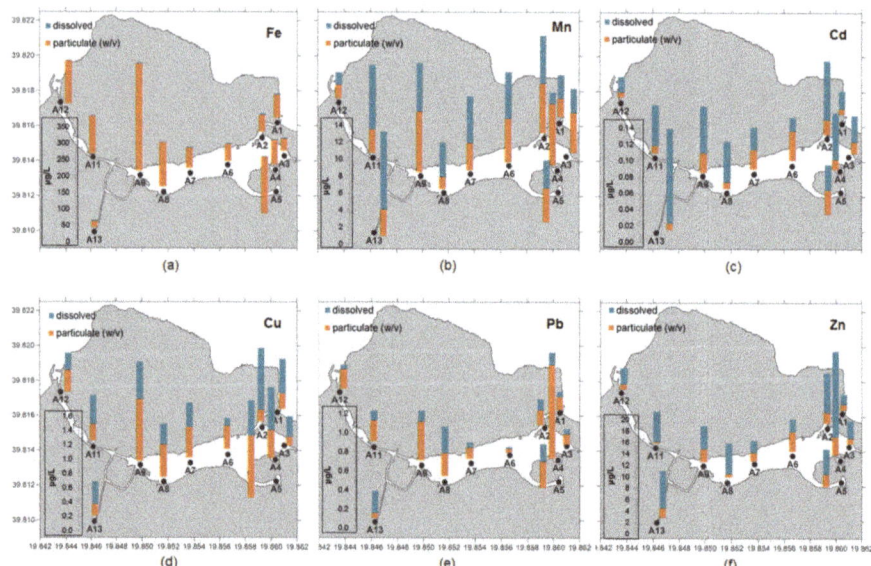

Figure 2. Spatial variation of dissolved and particulate (w/v) concentrations for (**a**) Fe, (**b**) Mn, (**c**) Cd, (**d**) Cu, (**e**) Pb, and (**f**) Zn.

Figure 3 illustrates the detailed distribution of particulate elements between the two fractions of suspended particles (d < 8 µm and >8 µm). The concentrations of particulate metals are expressed in w/w in order to compensate for differences of the SPM concentrations among the stations. Particles with d > 8 μm contained larger amounts of Al and Fe than the finer ones, of d < 8 μm. This distribution pattern is in contrast to the general and well established trend that as the grain size of particles decreases, the surface area increases, as does the particulate metal concentrations [36,37].

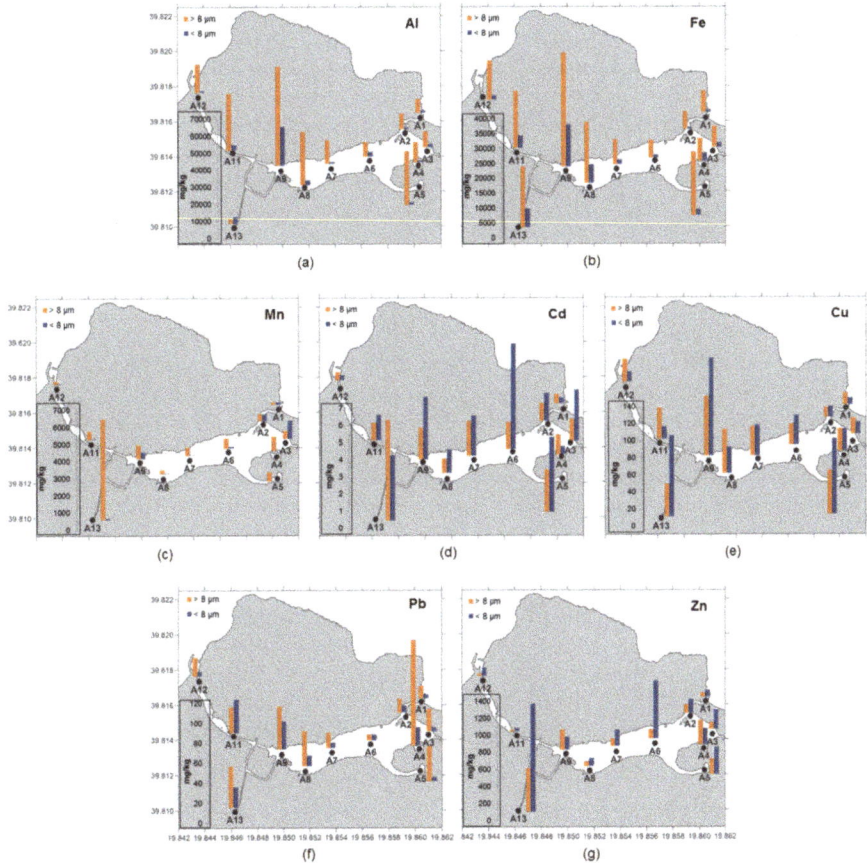

Figure 3. Spatial variation of particulate metal contents (w/w) of the >8 μm and the <8 μm fraction of SPM: (**a**) Al, (**b**) Fe, (**c**) Mn, (**d**) Cd, (**e**) Cu, (**f**) Pb, and (**g**) Zn.

The most probable explanation of the rather unusual, relative enrichment of larger particles is that these are agglomerated grains, consisting of aggregates of smaller particles [38] that are produced *in situ* through flocculation processes at the fresh-saline water interface [27,39,40]. The elevated Al, Fe, and Mn contents of the larger particles indicate that these phases are either: (a) linked to the original, smaller individual particulates, as a result of coagulation and precipitation of colloids and/or as surface coatings on clays [41]; or (b) that the newly formed agglomerates are cemented together by Fe/Mn coatings [37,38]. Some of the cement coatings could be organic in nature as well [37,42], since bacterially mediated processes may promote flocculation of smaller particles [43].

The presence of Al and Fe/Mn onto the larger particles increases their ability to sorb other metals. This is supported by the significant correlations between the elements in the > 8 μm fraction, shown in Table 2. Significant correlations of Cd, Cu, Pb, and Zn with Al, Fe, and Mn in the >8 μm fraction of SPM (r = 0.505–0.853; $\varrho < 0.05$) are consistent with the scavenging of metals by Al-Fe-Mn oxyhydroxides, and explains the enrichment with metals of the suspended particles >8 μm in relation to the finer particles

(<8 µm) (Figure 3). The strong correlation of suspended Pb with Al, Fe and Mn (r = 0.619–0.779) explains its predominant partitioning in all samplings and stations in the > 8 µm fractions of particles. Furthermore, the higher correlation coefficient of Pb and Fe over Al and Mn is compatible with its strong affinity (stability constant) for freshly precipitated Fe oxyhydroxides [32]. Cadmium and Zn correlated strongly with Mn (r = 0.949, and 0.710, respectively), suggesting the preferential association of these elements with Mn oxyhydroxides. According to Turner et al., [44] Cd binding onto Mn oxides is much stronger than on Fe oxyhydroxides or other phases.

The concentrations of particulate Mn, Cd, and Zn (in w/w) were significantly lower in the inlets than the inner part of the lagoon. This pattern suggests that these elements are entrapped within the lagoon. No statistical differences were determined for the other metals (Fe, Cu, Pb) between the inner sector and the inlets.

During the first sampling period, at the eastern inlet an inflow of relatively dense saline water (S: 37.2) near the bottom and an outflow of brackish water (S: 22.0) at the surface was evident from salinity measurements. An additional sample for trace metals and SPM determinations was collected from the near-bottom, saline layer at this site, to get insights into the processes occurring at this interface. Figure 4 shows the detailed distribution of particulate SPM, Al, Fe, and Mn between the two fractions of suspended particles (<8 µm and >8 µm) in the two water layers. SPM concentrations in the bottom, saline layer were higher (sum of both fractions: 41.9 mg·L^{-1}) than in the surface (13.4 mg·L^{-1}), suggesting the re-suspension of bottom sediments. The coarser fraction of SPM was the predominant one. Despite the re-suspension, the metal contents of the larger particles of the bottom water layer were slightly higher than those of the surface layer. Aluminum, Fe and Mn contents of the smaller particles were higher at the surface water layer than the bottom layer. Apparently, the flocculation and the enrichment mechanisms described above continued under the high salinity regime.

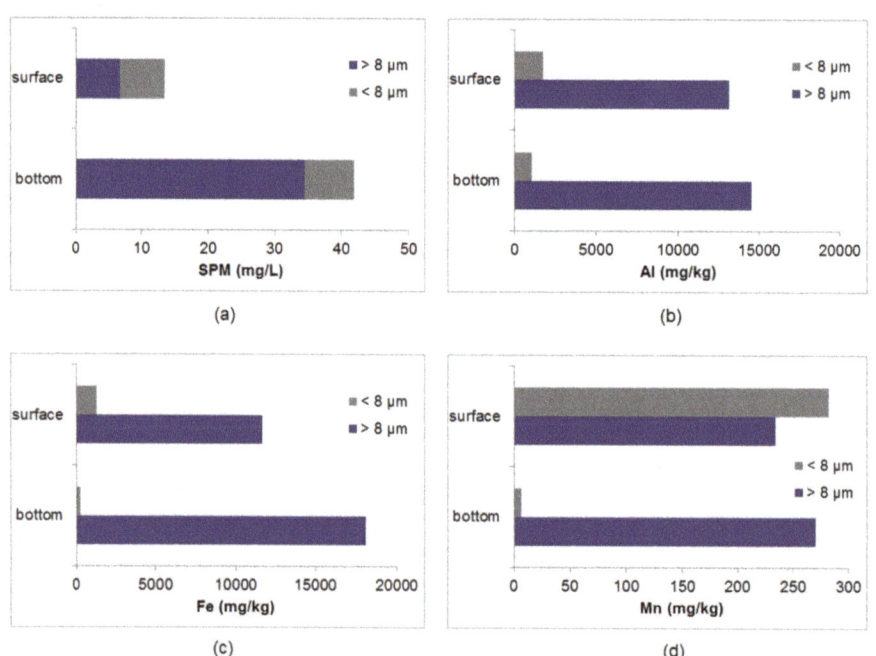

Figure 4. Concentrations of (**a**) SPM, and (**b**) Al, (**c**) Fe, and (**d**) Mn (w/w) contents of particulate solids with diameter d < 8 µm and d > 8 µm in the brackish surface and the saline bottom water layer of station A1.

4.2.2. Partitioning and Interactions between the Dissolved and Particulate Phases

According to Figure 2, in the inner part of the lagoon, Fe and Pb were primarily particle-bound (on average 94% and 70% of the total concentrations, respectively), Cd and Zn were found to be predominantly in the dissolved phase (67% and 70% of the total concentrations, respectively), whereas Cu and Mn were equally associated with the solid and solution phases. In the stream water, all elements were predominantly found in the dissolved phase, except Fe. The predominance of the dissolved phase for Mn and the particulate phase for Fe in stream water sample is compatible with the fact that oxidation kinetics of Mn(II), emanating from groundwater, is slower than that of Fe(II) [8,45].

Solid-solution partitioning of metals in estuarine systems has been widely described by the partition coefficient K_D, defined as [46]:

$$KD = \frac{\text{Particulate concentration} \left(\frac{w}{w}\right)}{\text{Dissolved concentration} \left(\frac{w}{v}\right)} \quad (1)$$

The partition coefficient should be constant for a given composition of suspended particles and of solution; however, any change of the particle surface reactivity and/or solution properties may result in K_D changes [47]. The partition coefficient is calculated in this study for all particles (K_{D-T}), for the large particles with diameter > 8 µm (K_{D-L}), and for the small particles with diameter d < 8 µm (K_{D-S}); (Table 3). This distinction allows the investigation of the role of each fraction of particles on the solid-solution partitioning in detail.

Table 3. Partition coefficient ($\log_{10}$) K_{D-T} for all the particles, K_{D-L} for particles with diameter d > 8 µm, and K_{D-S} for particles with 0.45 µm < d < 8 µm.

Partition Coefficient K_D	Statistics	Fe	Mn	Cd	Cu	Pb	Zn
K_{D-T}	mean	6.53	5.01	4.50	4.90	5.27	4.59
	min	5.74	4.51	3.59	3.86	4.86	3.76
	max	7.45	5.82	5.19	5.80	5.88	5.75
	mean inlets	6.51	4.89	4.11	4.63	5.23	4.30
	mean inner	6.57	4.99	4.68	4.94	5.33	4.65
	mean stream	6.40	5.43	4.62	5.42	5.11	5.03
K_{D-L}	mean	6.71	5.12	4.48	4.86	5.38	4.45
	min	5.95	4.58	3.60	3.88	4.93	3.67
	max	7.57	6.48	5.11	5.48	5.95	5.47
K_{D-S}	mean	5.77	4.16	4.52	4.89	4.91	4.55
	min	4.56	3.08	3.33	3.70	3.63	2.50
	max	7.10	5.87	5.45	5.86	5.67	5.81

The average K_{D-T} follows the order Fe < Pb < Mn < Cu < Zn, Cd (Table 3), and their values are similar to the ones reported for other transitional waters [48,49]. The elevated K_{D-T} values for Fe and Pb indicate these metals are associated with and transported in the particulate phase, whereas the low K_{D-T} values for Zn and Cd confirm their affinity to the dissolved phase.

The values of K_{D-L} for the large particles were, in general, higher than the K_{D-S} values for the smaller ones. This is consistent with the removal from solution through flocculation of Fe and Mn and co-precipitation processes for trace metals, resulting in elevated metal contents of the large particles (Figures 3 and 4). Figure 5 illustrates the variation of K_D values for Cd, Zn, and Cu with salinity in the inner part of the lagoon (n = 10). These plots are advantageous to the widely used metals concentrations/salinity relationships because they allow for the exchange processes between the dissolved and particulate phases to be considered [49]. The K_{D-S} values for Cd and Zn decreased with increasing salinity (r = −0.869; ϱ = 0.001 and r = −0.740; ϱ = 0.013, respectively), but not the K_{D-L}. These results show that the exchange processes take place predominantly between the smaller fraction of

SPM (<8 μm) and the dissolved phase, rather the coarser fraction of SPM (>8 μm). The lack of a clear relationship of the K_{D-L} values for Cd and Zn with salinity could be attributed to their strong binding to Mn oxyhydroxides of the large particles (Table 2). Turner et.al. [44] showed that, when Cd is bound to Mn oxides, it is less prone to desorption across the salinity gradient. In contrast, the decrease of the K_{D-S} values with increasing salinity could be attributed to desorption. In the case of Cd, this behavior is often attributed in the formation of highly stable and soluble chloro-complexes [1,50,51]. As far as Cu is concerned, both K_{D-S} and the K_{D-L} values decreased with increasing salinity, suggesting the removal of both SPM fractions to the solution. The non-conservative behavior of Cu has been ascribed in more detailed studies to the strong Cu-complexing ligands such as organic colloids and dissolved organic matter [52,53]. Dissolved Cu concentrations did not vary between the inner part and the inlets of the lagoon. Thus, it can be suggested that desorption from the solid phase enhances the dispersion of dissolved Cu beyond the boundaries of the lagoon.

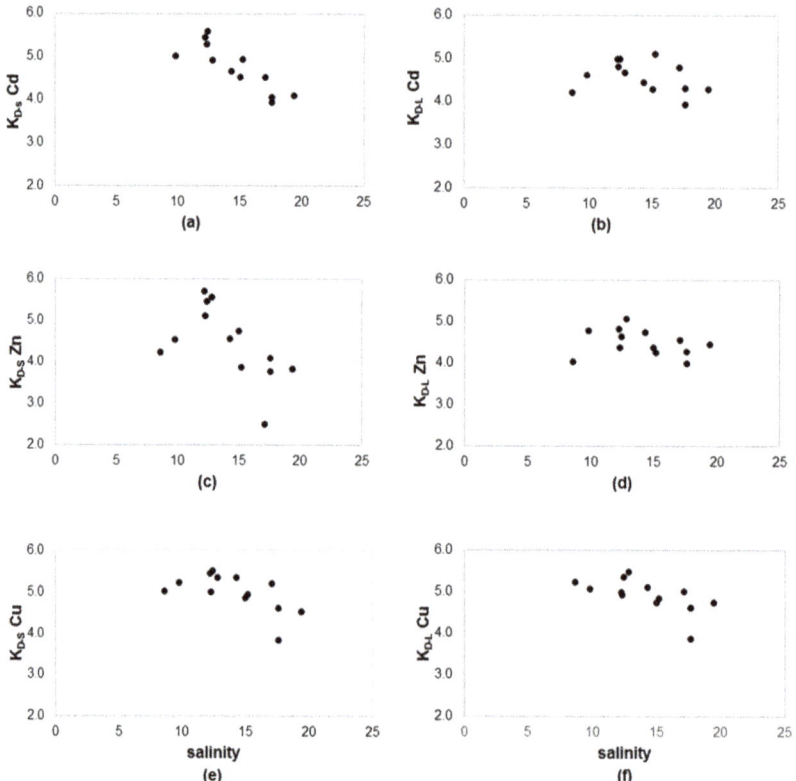

Figure 5. Variation of partition coefficient (K_D) with salinity the inner part of the lagoon: (**a**) K_{D-S} for Cd of the small particles (<8 μm) (**b**) K_{D-L} for Cd of the large particles (d < 8 μm), (**c**) K_{D-S} for Zn, and (**d**) K_{D-L} for Zn, (**e**) K_{D-S} for Cu, and (**f**) K_{D-L} for Cu.

4.3. Surface Sediments

Organic carbon content in the silt and clay fraction (<63 μm) of the surficial sediments of two inlets was low and ranged from 0.26% to 0.59%, whereas at the inner part and the outlet of the stream it ranged between 3.97%–8.20%, and 10.40%, respectively (Table 4). Organic-rich sediments are common in coastal lagoons [14], mainly due to the high productivity of these systems in relation to other coastal marine and estuarine systems.

Table 4. Organic carbon (OC in %), total (T in mg·kg^{-1}) and 0.5 N HCl extractable (Ext in mg·kg^{-1}) metal contents in the surficial and core sediments.

Sampling Stations/ Statistics	OC	Al-T	Fe-T	Fe-Ext	Mn-T	Mn-Ext	Cd-T	Cd-Ext	Cu-T	Cu-Ext	Pb-T	Pb-Ext	Zn-T	Zn-Ext
						Surface Sediments								
A1	0.26	11000	3130	1260	350	330	0.14	0.08	12	2.04	4.05	2.04	9.23	5.36
A2	4.32	25000	10700	4980	190	150	0.69	0.45	25	13.9	31.8	23.9	50.4	27.4
A3	5.92	30100	12100	4370	140	73	1.89	1.09	32	18.7	29.3	23.7	75.1	36.4
A4	8.52	31100	18200	3630	170	68	2.04	1.79	41	37.6	33.1	31.9	89.2	56.9
A5	10.6	39300	20800	5140	200	66	3.42	3.12	50	22.4	66.1	49.6	106	49.7
A7	4.78	62600	30800	4930	310	153	1.66	1.02	56	23.8	23.1	18.9	121	47.4
A8	7.79	48000	24000	8910	180	75	1.71	1.02	57	28.6	36.5	25.8	122	46.4
A9	3.97	28800	17500	10760	170	150	0.22	0.17	32	17.9	22.9	18.5	72.5	31.1
A10	11.2	41900	31700	14200	330	210	0.43	0.41	75	42.4	25.3	23.1	98.4	55.2
A12	0.59	9790	3800	1980	150	140	0.17	0.05	13	3.10	8.29	2.33	17.2	8.80
A13	10.4	33900	20100	10100	210	190	0.59	0.48	37	20.6	25.3	19.4	70.8	32.2
Mean	6.2	32800	17500	6390	220	150	1.18	0.88	39	21.0	27.8	21.7	75.6	37.2
Median	5.9	31100	18200	4980	200	150	0.69	0.48	37	20.6	25.3	23.1	75.1	36.4
Min	0.3	9790	3130	1260	140	66	0.14	0.05	12	2.04	4.05	2.04	9.23	9.23
Max	11.2	62500	31700	14200	350	330	3.42	3.12	75	42.4	66.1	49.6	121.7	56.9
Sd	3.8	15300	9520	4050	73	80	1.05	0.91	20	12.4	16.1	13.0	37.8	15.5
						Core Sediments								
Mean	7.3	56900	24000	7406	129	33.4	1.47	1.24	57	28.0	74.4	48.2	143	39.6
Median	6.9	49800	21600	5713	123	21.1	0.81	0.64	58	28.9	40.4	28.8	141	41.6
Min	2.4	33500	19300	1762	105	11.7	0.23	0.19	36	18.6	19.9	8.13	91.1	27.3
Max	11.9	90200	40300	21276	178	88.4	3.51	2.97	69	32.9	566	300	202	53.2
Sd	3.3	17400	5800	5631	19.0	25.2	1.17	1.08	9.4	4.15	113	62.9	28.6	8.38

Total metals contents in the surface sediments followed the order (median values): Al (33100 mg·kg^{-1}) > Fe (18200 mg·kg^{-1}) > Mn (200 mg·kg^{-1}) > Zn (75 mg·kg^{-1}) > Cu (37.0 mg·kg^{-1}) > Pb (25.3 mg·kg^{-1}) Cd > 0.69 mg·kg^{-1}), and varied widely on the spatial scale (Table 4). Aluminum, the structural component of clay minerals, ranged from 6790 to 62,500 mg·kg^{-1}. The lower Al values were determined at the two inlets, due to the high abundance of carbonates and quartz at these sediments. The higher ones were determined at the central part of the lagoon (stations A7, A8), as well as the outlet of the stream (station A10), indicating the preferable accumulation of terrigenous aluminosilicates at these sites.

The large variation of Al contents suggests that granulometric and mineralogical differences exist among the sediment samples. This is despite the fact that sieving out the sand fraction provides theoretically a more homogeneous fraction of the sediment for metal levels estimation and distribution patterns analysis. Thus, normalization to Al was employed in order to further minimize grain-size effects [15,28].

Figure 6 shows the spatial variation of metal to Al (Me/Al) ratios. The highest Fe/Al values were observed at the outlet of the stream, whereas the lowest ones at the two inlets. A similar distribution pattern is observed for Cu. Copper correlated with Al (r = 0.936; ϱ < 0.0005) and Fe (r = 0.982; ϱ < 0.0005), suggesting their common transport pathway through land run-off and a similar deposition pattern in the surface sediments. Cadmium to Al, as well as Pb/Al ratio values were higher at the eastern part of the lagoon and exhibited maxima at the sediments of station A4. Values of Zn/Al were rather homogeneous throughout the lagoon, however, a local maximum was observed at station A4. Zinc correlated with Al (r = 0.918; ϱ < 0.0005) and Fe (r = 0.918; ϱ < 0.0005), which is indicative of their common origin from terrestrial sources.

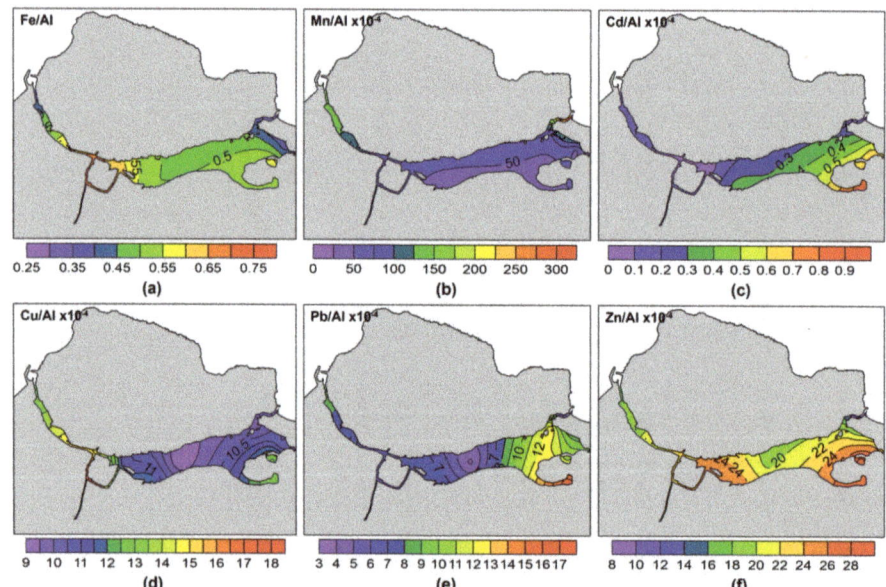

Figure 6. Spatial distribution of (**a**) Fe/Al, (**b**) Mn/Al, (**c**) Cd/Al, (**d**) Cu/Al, (**e**) Pb/Al, and (**f**) Zn/Al values in the surface sediments of the Antinioti Lagoon.

The potential mobility of metals under changing environmental conditions, thus their (bio)availability, can be estimated by extracting the sediment samples with dilute HCl (0.5 N) [54]. The procedure extracts the fraction of metals retained in sediments by adsorption, complexation and precipitation processes [55].

The extractability of metals (i.e., the percentage of 0.5 HCl extracted contents in relation to total contents) in the surface sediments followed the order (median value): Fe (40%) < Zn (48%) < Cu (56%) < Mn, Cd (65%) < Pb (77%), suggesting that Fe and Zn were the most inert metals, whereas Pb, Cd and Mn the potentially more mobile metals under changing environmental conditions. The extractability of Mn at the sediments of the two inlets and the stream accounted for more than 90%. This substantial increase of the extractability in the inlets and the stream compared to the inner part of the lagoon (median value: 51%) suggests that in the former areas Mn is found in more labile phases, which are related to the flocculation processes discussed previously.

Dilute HCl extractable Cd, Cu, Pb and Zn contents were significantly correlated with OC content (r = 0.629–0.827; ϱ < 0.05), which is consistent with the findings of Yuan et al. [42]. The association of this fraction of metals with OC may result in the mobilization of metals along with the oxidation of OC. [8,18]. More insights into diagenetic processes are gained through the examination of core sediments.

4.4. Core Sediments

Organic carbon content varied widely with depth and ranged from 2.4% to 11.9% (Figure 7). The lower values found in the sediments below 25 cm depth, indicate the decomposition of organic matter with time, while the higher values found within the 4–20 cm sediment interval imply buried organic matter not yet degraded [56]. High OC contents result in high oxygen consumption and, subsequently, in the establishment of sub-oxic, anoxic, and/or sulfidic conditions in the sub-surface sediments. Black-gray bands and dots were observed within the 6–24 cm sediment interval, which indicate the presence of sulfides. Deeper in the sediment column, in the 24–31 cm interval, sediments had a reddish-brown color that indicates the presence of iron oxyhydroxides [45,57].

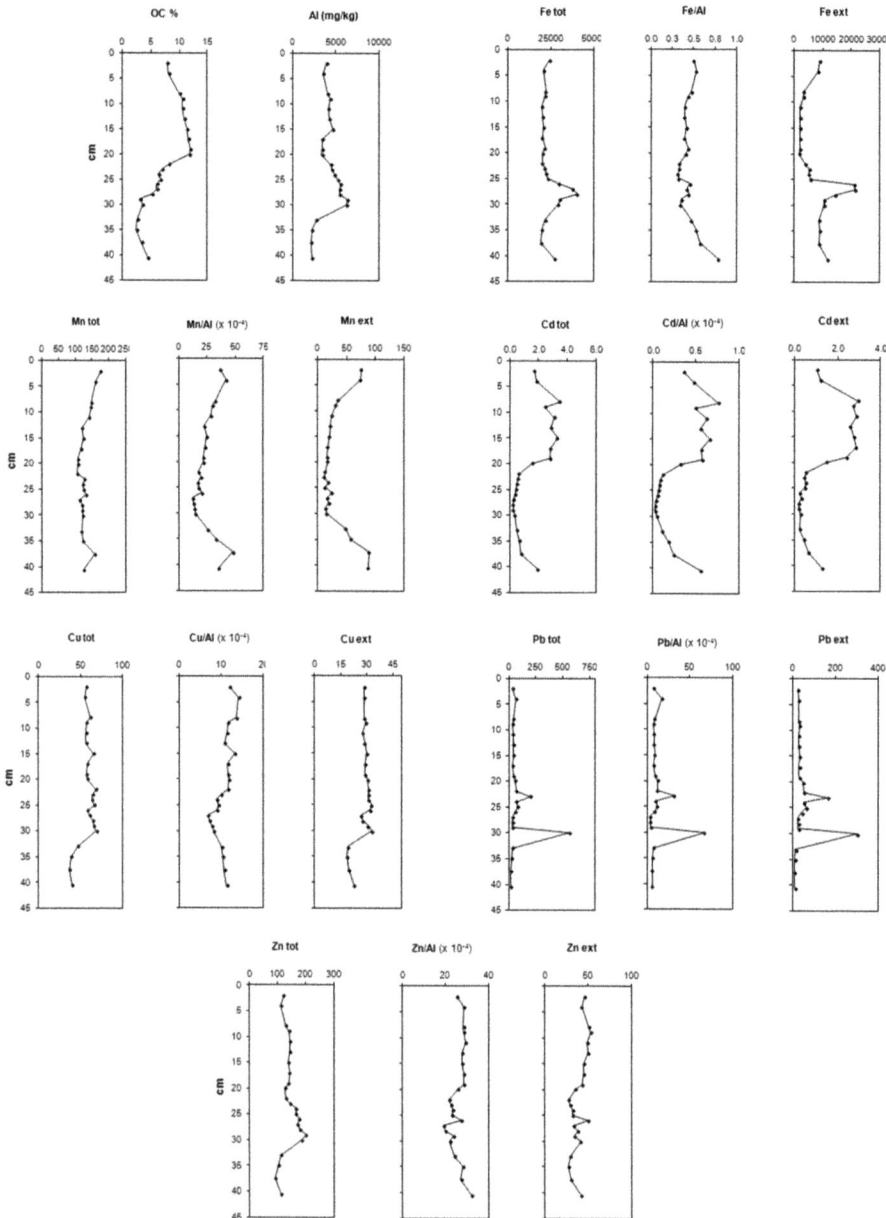

Figure 7. Vertical distributions of total, 0.5N HCl extractable, and normalized to Al metal contents in the core sediments.

The levels of Al, Fe, Cd, Cu and Zn in the core sediments were similar to those found in the surficial ones, whereas the levels of Mn were slightly lower (Table 4). The extractability of metals by 0.5 N HCl in the core sediments followed the order (median): Mn (17%) < Fe (25%) < Zn (28%) < Cu (49%) < Pb (71%) < Cd (83%). The lower percentages of extracted metals, particularly for Mn and Fe, compared to the surface sediments, signify their presence in different forms. This could be attributed to: (a) the processes occurring in the water column that involve the complexation of metals with organic and inorganic ligands and the formation of metal precipitates; and (b) the processes occurring in the sediment column that involve the redistribution of metals on the geochemical substrates, or even a partial release from the sediments to the water column, triggered by diagenetic redox processes.

The extractability of Mn by the dilute HCl decreased from 44% of the total content at the surface layer to less than 20% within the 9–30 cm sediment interval. The profile of 0.5N HCl extracted Mn (Figure 7) shows an increasing trend from the depth of 30 cm towards the surface, which is typical of the progressive dissolution of Mn oxyhydroxides, upward diffusion of at least part of Mn(II) dissolved ions, and re-oxidation/precipitation at the surface layer where higher redox potentials are met [58]. With this process, the least labile fraction of Mn is left behind, thus the extractability of Mn is lower in the subsurface sediments than in the surficial ones.

The amount of Fe extracted by the dilute HCl varied widely with depth from 9% to 71% of the total Fe content. The highest percentages coincide with the observed orange- bands, which are attributed to accumulations of Fe oxyhydroxides that are fully recovered by the extractant [59]; the lower percentages coincide with the black-grey bands, which could signify the presence of pyrite, the end-product of metastable Fe-monosulfides with hydrogen sulfide [60], which are not extracted by HCl [59]. Previous research at the site [23] confirmed the presence of pyrite in the subsurface sediments of the Antinioti Lagoon by means of X-ray Diffraction and Scanning Electron Microscope analysis. However, within the pyritized sediments, micro-environments of authigenic Fe/Mn oxides (Mn containing goethite) were identified through synchrotron radiation micro X-ray fluorescence (SR µ-XRF).

Total and 0.5 N HCl extracted Cd contents were significantly correlated with OC content (r = 0.695 and 0.783, respectively; $\varrho < 0.0005$). The profiles were similar to each other and showed lower contents near the water-sediment interface, a substantial increase in the 4–20 cm sediments layers, followed by a further decrease after this depth. This distribution pattern has been described in previous studies [19,58], and is consistent with Cd dissolution after the oxic degradation near the surface of fresh organic carbon with which Cd was originally bound, and downward diffusion and fixation, in the thick zone of sub-oxic to anoxic grey-black colored, underlying sediments, which are depleted in Mn. This pattern is typical in sub-oxic sediments where authigenic accumulations, as CdS precipitates, take place [19,58,61,62]. Cadmium sulfide minerals are fully recovered by HCl [63], and this explains the high amounts of Cd extracted by the procedure (median value: 85%) in relation to the total metal.

The vertical distribution of total and 0.5 N HCl-extracted Pb is dominated by two extreme values at 23 cm (203 and 161 mg·kg^{-1}, respectively) and 30 cm (566 and 300 mg·kg^{-1}, respectively). These peaks are most probably attributed to distinct and occasional events of pollution, which are unknown to us.

4.5. Enrichment Factors

The magnitude and spatial extent of human-induced change was determined by expressing current normalized to Al metal contents as enrichment over pre-anthropogenic or background levels through the widely used Enrichment Factor (EF) [53,64]. The EF is estimated according to the formula:

$$EF = \frac{(\text{element}/\text{Al})\text{sample}}{(\text{element}/\text{Al})\text{background}} \quad (2)$$

For the calculation of the local background levels, the median elements values of the deeper part (30–37.5 cm) of the core were used. The sedimentation rate in the lagoon, estimated in another core obtained from station A4 by ^{210}Pb analysis, is 0.3 cm·y^{-1} [23]. Thus, the 30–37.5 cm sediments interval corresponds to accumulations more than 100-years old, i.e., well before the urbanization of the study area. Additionally, those sediments had a light brown color, are thus considered as being oxic, and no apparent authigenic accumulations were observed. The metal contents used as the local background were: 38 mg·kg^{-1} for Cu, 104 mg·kg^{-1} for Zn, 25 mg·kg^{-1} for Pb and 0.69 mg·kg^{-1} for Cd. These values are similar to the upper boundaries of the 2N HCl extractable metal contents reported by Voutsinou-Taliadouri [65] at the unpolluted, Kerkyra strait, i.e., the marine area between the island and NW Greece: 3–30 mg·kg^{-1} for Cu, 7–24 mg·kg^{-1} for Pb and 21–94 mg·kg^{-1} for Zn. Therefore, the levels proposed here are considered as the best approximation of the local background levels.

Interestingly, the local background for Cd is twice higher than the average shale (0.3 mg· kg^{-1}) reported by Turekian and Wedepohl, [66], and almost 8 times higher than the value of upper continental crust (0.09 mg·kg^{-1}) [67]. A possible reason for this discrepancy is that phosphate bearing limestones, which outcrop in Kerkyra Island, have been found to contain significant amounts of Cd as impurities [68].

Enrichment factors of 1.5–3, 3–5, 5–10 and >10 times are classified as minor, moderate, severe and very severe modification, respectively [69]. The median values of EFs for the anthropogenic metals were low, falling within the range of minor contamination (Cu: 1.1; Zn: 0.9; Pb: 0.9; Cd: 1.4). However, the maximum values of EF for Cd (5.7 at station A5; 3.5 at station A4; and 3.4 at station A3; see elevated Cd/Al values in Figure 6), indicate moderate anthropogenic modification, confined in localized areas of the lagoon. There are no industries located at the wider area of the lagoon that could explain this enrichment. Considering the land uses of the Antinioti drainage basin, Cd may partly derive from phosphate fertilizers that are applied in the adjacent cultivated areas. Another possible source of these metals could be the leaching of solid wastes improperly disposed at the riparian area. Nevertheless, the incidence of high levels in sediments, the suspended matter and the dissolved phase close to the freshwater seepage sites (e.g., A5, A8, A13), complicates further the source apportionment. So far, our results suggest that the freshwater inputs contribute significantly to Cd contamination. Yet, it is unclear whether the percolating water through the karstic formations becomes enriched by anthropogenic activities throughout its flow path prior to its discharge into the lagoon, or it becomes enriched by leaching of bedrock, or other complex geochemical processes.

In the core sediments, EFs ranges were 0.7–1.4 for Cu, 0.7–1.2 for Zn, 0.1–4.1 for Cd and 0.6–10 for Pb. The vertical distributions of EFs, i.e., the evolution of contamination, are similar to the profiles of elemental ratios to Al shown in Figure 7. The highest EF values for Pb were recorded at distinct sediment layers, consistent with the distinct contamination events discussed previously. The highest EF values for Cd correspond to the thick sediment layer at the top 20 cm of the core that is influenced by diagenetic alterations; thus this should not be attributed entirely to contamination. The values of EF for Cu and Zn, remained low and rather constant in time.

5. Discussion

Antinioti Lagoon is a remote, shallow, non-industrialized and not particularly urbanized system that has a high biodiversity and is of major geochemical interest. The present assessment of heavy metals in the various compartments of this lagoonal system provides a series of conclusions and raises some critical issues to be addressed in forthcoming research projects that will be discussed hereafter.

The freshwater spring of groundwater origin that flows as a stream into the lagoon, is the major source of dissolved Mn, Cd, and Pb, as well as particulate (w/w) Mn, Cd, and Zn (Table 2). The importance of groundwater discharges as a transport pathway of nutrients, carbon, and trace metals has been acknowledged in other coastal lagoon settings [7,70] and they are considered as a rival contributor to riverine inputs of land-derived material into the ocean [45,71,72]. Groundwater seepage in the Antinioti Lagoon is a field for future research, in order to elucidate whether the enrichment ascribes to natural geochemical processes, i.e., diagenesis, or to anthropogenic activities (e.g., the use of Cd- bearing phosphate fertilizers) throughout its catchment area.

Trace metals participate in a series of critical, physical and geochemical processes that define their mobility and fate within the transitional fresh-saline water interface and beyond. Precipitation of Al, Fe, Mn oxyhydroxides, and flocculation are probably the most important ones. These processes are considered to be responsible for the rather unusual enrichment of large (> 8 μm) particles, both at the stream and within the lagoon (Figure 3). Precipitates of clays and Fe/Mn oxyhydroxides on large suspended solids (>8 μm), probably as composite coatings with organic matter, strongly affect the ability of this fraction of SPM to bind trace metals. Scavenging of Pb predominantly by Fe oxyhydroxides, Cd and Zn by Mn oxyhydroxides and Cu by Al and Fe/Mn phases explains the enrichment of the coarser particles (>8 μm) with metals in relation to the finer ones (<8 μm). Furthermore, the large particles were found to be less prone to desorption processes than the smaller ones. With increasing salinity, the partition coefficient of the small particles for Cd, and Zn decreased, as a result of desorption. In contrast, the variability of K_{D-L} values was much smaller (Figure 5).

Scavenging of trace metals by large particles, with higher settling velocities than the finer ones, has serious implications on their transport and dispersion patterns across the system. Although the density of flocs is unknown and particle settling rates cannot be accurately estimated, in the grain-size range of 1–100 μm, the settling velocity of grains of ~100 μm is in the order of 10^4 larger than the settling velocity of particles of 1 μm [73]. Thus, the enrichment mechanism of large particles with metals, combined with the irreversible adsorption of Cd and Zn onto Mn oxyhydroxides may explain the efficient entrapment of Mn, Cd, and Zn within the boundaries of the lagoon, evidenced by their significantly lower particulate concentrations (w/w) in the inlets than in the inner part. The behavior of Cu was differentiated from Cd, and Zn in the way that desorption occurred from both fractions of SPM, causing the dispersal of Cu in the dissolved phase beyond the system. According to Roussiez et al., [53] the removal of Cu into solution was not restricted in the fresh-saline water interface but instead, continued well after the deposition of fluvial material through the degradation of organic matter with which Cu was originally bound.

Resuspension of bottom sediments is expected to cause a decrease of particulate trace metal contents due to the mixing of enriched brackish water particles with high trace metal contents with coarse particles with low metal contents of marine origin [74]; this was not the case in our study. Aluminum, Fe, and Mn contents of the coarser fraction of the SPM in the bottom saline water were higher than in the surface layer, despite the resuspension of sediments (Figure 4). Such an enrichment is attributed to flocculation processes occurring at high salinity regimes. Sholkovitz [75], with a series of laboratory experiments, showed that although the amount of flocculated Al is maximized at salinity 12, at higher salinities the removal of Al from solution reaches a constant value. In the case of Mn, its removal from the solution increases and levels off at salinities 15–25, whereas an additional removal occurs at salinities 27–30. At the same time, the finer fraction of SPM increased at the surface layer. The presence of fine-grained particles in suspension has been described by Eisma [73] as re-flocculation observed in several estuarine systems. According to the latter author, at the saline part of the estuary, flocs of fluvial origin are broken up by organisms that consume the organic matter gluing the particles together. Re-suspension of organic matter will then result in newly formed flocs with organic matter of estuarine origin. Although the exact mechanism is not known, flocculation at the seaward boundary of transitional water systems may have serious implications on the transport and dispersion of pollutants across a system, as suggested by previous studies [53,76–78].

In the sediments, the occasionally elevated values of EF for Cd and Pb, falling within the range of moderate modification in the surface sediments to severe modification in the core sediments, prioritize these elements in terms of environmental concern and pollution abatement measures. The labile fractions of Cu, Cd, Pb and Zn in the surface sediments were found to be associated with organic matter. Future studies should consider the analysis of planktonic samples to further elucidate the role of organic matter in the transport and accumulation of trace elements in the sediments. Nevertheless, the high organic carbon content in the core sediments (up to 12%) has been shown to influence the post-depositional distribution of total and labile fractions of metals. Accumulations of Cd coinciding with Mn depletions in gray-black sub-surface sediments, suggest that the profiles of these elements are greatly influenced by diagenetic processes.

Looking to the future, decision making should balance the sustainability of values and functions of the lagoon and the risks associated to the remobilization potential of toxic trace elements from the sediments. Dredging of sediments for the maintenance of the fish overwintering trench could result in the oxidation of sub-surface sediments, with high potential of releasing significant amounts of metals that would pose consequent environmental risks for the biota as well as economic and health risks for the end consumers.

Author Contributions: Conceptualization, F.B. and M.S.; methodology, F.B.; software, F.B. and A.K.; validation, F.B. and V.P.; formal analysis, F.B.; investigation, F.B., V.P.; resources, M.D. and M.S.; writing—original draft preparation, F.B.; writing—review and editing, F.B., A.K., M.S.; visualization, F.B. and A.K.; supervision, M.S.; project administration, F.B.; funding acquisition, M.S. and M.D.

Funding: This research received no external funding.

Acknowledgments: We wish to thank Eleftheria Aperi, Olga Chalkiadaki and Paraskevi Skourti for their valuable help in the laboratory. We also thank people in the Kerkyra Island for providing assistance in the field and useful information about the study area.

Conflicts of Interest: The authors declare no conflict of interest.

Appendix A

Table A1. Detailed results of salinity, pH, Suspended Particulate Matter (SPM in mg·L^{-1}) and dissolved (d. in µg·L^{-1}), total (dissolved and particulate, t., in µg·L^{-1}) and particulate (p. in mg·kg^{-1}) metal concentrations of the 1st and 2nd sampling campaigns.

Sampling Stations	Salinity	pH	SPM	p.Al	t.Fe	d.Fe	p.Fe	t.Mn	d.Mn	p.Mn	t.Cd	d.Cd	p.Cd	t.Cu	d.Cu	p.Cu	t.Pb	d.Pb	p.Pb	t.Zn	d.Zn	p.Zn
										1st sampling campaign												
A1 surf.	22.0	8.0	13.4	7517	94.1	6.36	6571	7.80	4.36	258	0.030	0.019	0.78	0.54	0.31	16.9	0.18	0.06	9.6	2.63	1.2	107
A1 bott.	37.2	7.9	41.9	12195	633	7.19	14949	10.2	0.81	224	0.028	0.018	0.23	0.69	0.30	9.10	0.62	0.15	11.3	6.60	3.13	82.8
A2	15.0	8.2	14.2	6452	56.1	6.32	3496	14.5	6.98	531	0.099	0.073	1.83	0.37	0.20	12.3	0.21	0.07	10.0	7.72	5.03	189
A3	12.3	7.7	7.5	6219	37.2	5.91	4162	9.54	2.86	889	0.051	0.028	3.06	0.18	0.11	9.88	0.12	0.05	9.2	4.87	3.33	205
A5	12.2	7.5	8.1	6335	32.8	1.23	3899	6.85	4.42	301	0.061	0.027	4.20	0.35	0.16	24.1	0.11	0.02	10.4	3.19	1.23	243
A7	12.8	8.2	12.4	7818	62.7	2.93	4833	7.12	4.29	229	0.067	0.039	2.30	0.41	0.09	25.4	0.13	0.03	8.3	3.43	1.00	197
A9	9.8	7.8	9.8	15103	95.5	2.40	10032	10.1	7.13	316	0.057	0.036	2.23	0.34	0.15	20.6	0.21	0.03	19.5	3.02	2.01	108
A12	37.7	8.1	14.9	6787	92.5	3.58	5981	3.01	1.71	87	0.030	0.019	0.70	0.49	0.18	20.7	0.20	0.03	11.2	5.18	3.67	102
A13	4.7	7.5	1.5	4204	12.9	2.61	6731	5.89	2.91	1945	0.077	0.069	5.23	0.31	0.16	101	0.25	0.20	36.9	5.91	3.17	1790
										2nd sampling campaign												
A1	30.0	8.2	20.9	2432	50.4	0.66	2379	3.09	1.12	35.9	0.027	0.025	0.09	0.87	0.66	6.67	0.21	0.06	7.04	3.09	2.64	21.4
A2	17.6	8.0	13.8	4905	56.0	2.09	3923	10.0	4.20	301	0.081	0.071	0.69	1.68	1.53	11.1	0.34	0.17	12.4	10.0	8.99	80.7
A3	19.4	7.9	7.0	6776	42.9	1.03	5948	3.32	nm	407	0.041	0.037	0.63	0.63	0.47	22.9	0.15	nm	21.5	3.32	2.89	70.3
A5	17.1	7.5	13.2	32855	314	1.87	23572	9.82	2.15	419	0.059	0.035	1.81	2.37	0.83	105	0.81	0.34	35.2	9.82	7.62	212
A7	15.2	8.3	10.3	9091	63.3	0.42	6102	3.58	6.84	350	0.036	0.017	1.84	1.13	0.59	46.8	0.21	0.08	13.0	3.58	3.15	49.6
A9	14.3	8.0	10.5	90457	566	2.08	58612	9.42	4.31	1213	0.105	0.079	3.17	2.44	0.90	177	0.84	0.21	68.2	9.42	6.06	424
A12	37.5	8.2	14.3	15629	175	0.43	11996	2.24	1.23	131	0.019	0.018	0.09	0.62	0.30	22.1	0.30	0.06	16.5	2.24	2.06	11.9
A13	4.8	7.5	2.0	3406	30.1	5.23	12793	10.5	15.4	1667	0.171	0.164	3.76	0.64	0.47	51.3	0.31	0.27	22.9	10.5	9.94	198

Table 2. Spearman correlation coefficient (r) of particulate elements (w/w) in the > 8 μm fraction of particulates and significance level (ϱ)

Variable	Correlation Coefficient	Al	Fe	Mn	Cu	Cd	Zn	Pb
Al	r	-	0.844 **	0.153	0.744 **	0.042	0.086	0.619 **
	ϱ	-	0.000	0.533	0.000	0.864	0.726	0.005
Fe	r	0.844 **	-	0.364	0.853 **	0.209	0.179	0.779 **
	ϱ	0.000	-	0.115	0.000	0.376	0.450	0.000
Mn	r	0.153	0.364	-	0.505 *	0.649 **	0.710 **	0.633 **
	ϱ	0.533	0.115	-	0.023	0.002	0.000	0.003
Cu	r	0.744 **	0.853 **	0.505 *	-	0.372	0.197	0.732 **
	ϱ	0.000	0.000	0.023	-	0.107	0.405	0.000
Cd	r	0.042	0.209	0.649 **	0.372	-	0.601 **	0.256
	ϱ	0.864	0.376	0.002	0.107	-	0.005	0.276
Zn	r	0.086	0.179	0.710 **	0.197	0.601 **	-	0.395
	ϱ	0.726	0.450	0.000	0.405	0.005	-	0.084
Pb	r	0.619 **	0.779 **	0.633 **	0.732 **	0.256	0.395	-
	ϱ	0.005	0.000	0.003	0.000	0.276	0.084	-

** Correlation is significant at the 0.01 level (2-tailed); * Correlation is significant at the 0.05 level (2-tailed).

References

1. Martin, J.-M.; Huang, W.W.; Yoon, Y.Y. Level and fate of trace metals in the lagoon of Venice (Italy). *Mar. Chem.* **1994**, *46*, 371–386. [CrossRef]
2. Loureiro, D.D.; Fernandez, M.A.; Herms, F.W.; Lacerda, L.D. Heavy metal inputs evolution to an urban hypertrophic coastal lagoon, Rodrigo De Freitas Lagoon, Rio De Janeiro, Brazil. *Environ. Monit. Assess.* **2009**, *159*, 577. [CrossRef] [PubMed]
3. Accornero, A.; Gnerre, R.; Manfra, L. Sediment concentrations of trace metals in the Berre Lagoon (France): An assessment of contamination. *Arch. Environ. Contam. Toxicol.* **2008**, *54*, 372–385. [CrossRef] [PubMed]
4. Beltrame, M.O.; De Marco, S.G.; Marcovecchio, J.E. Dissolved and particulate heavy metals distribution in coastal lagoons. A case study from Mar Chiquita Lagoon, Argentina. *Estuar. Coast. Shelf Sci.* **2009**, *85*, 45–56. [CrossRef]
5. Karageorgis, A.P.; Sioulas, A.; Krasakopoulou, E.; Anagnostou, C.L.; Hatiris, G.A.; Kyriakidou, H.; Vasilopoulos, K. Geochemistry of surface sediments and heavy metal contamination assessment: Messolonghi Lagoon complex, Greece. *Environ. Earth Sci.* **2012**, *65*, 1619–1629. [CrossRef]
6. Uluturhan, E.; Kontas, A.; Can, E. Sediment concentrations of heavy metals in the Homa Lagoon (Eastern Aegean Sea): Assessment of contamination and ecological risks. *Mar. Pollut. Bull.* **2011**, *62*, 1989–1997. [CrossRef] [PubMed]
7. Kharroubi, A.; Gzam, M.; Jedoui, Y. Anthropogenic and natural effects on the water and sediments qualities of costal lagoons: Case of the Boughrara Lagoon (Southeast Tunisia). *Environ. Earth Sci.* **2012**, *67*, 1061–1067. [CrossRef]
8. Santos-Echeandia, J.; Prego, R.; Cobelo-García, A.; Millward, G.E. Porewater geochemistry in a galician ria (NW Iberian Peninsula): Implications for benthic fluxes of dissolved trace elements (Co, Cu, Ni, Pb, V, Zn). *Mar. Chem.* **2009**, *117*, 77–87. [CrossRef]
9. Point, D.; Monperrus, M.; Tessier, E.; Chauvaud, L.; Thouzeau, G.; Jean, F.; Amice, E.; Grall, J.; Leynaert, A.; Clavier, J.; et al. Biological control of trace metal and organometal benthic fluxes in a eutrophic lagoon (Thau Lagoon, Mediterranean Sea, France). *Estuar. Coast. Shelf Sci.* **2007**, *72*, 457–471. [CrossRef]
10. Turner, A.; Millward, G.E.; Le Roux, S.M. Significance of oxides and particulate organic matter in controlling trace metal partitioning in a contaminated estuary. *Mar. Chem.* **2004**, *88*, 179–192. [CrossRef]
11. Zwolsman, J.J.; van Eck, G.T. Geochemistry of major elements and trace metals in suspended matter of the Scheldt Estuary, Southwest Netherlands. *Mar. Chem.* **1999**, *66*, 91–111. [CrossRef]

12. Scoullos, M.; Botsou, F. Geochemical processes of trace metals in fresh–saline water interfaces. The cases of Louros and Acheloos estuaries. In *The Rivers of Greece: Evolution, Current Status and Perspectives*; Skoulikidis, N., Dimitriou, E., Karaouzas, I., Eds.; Springer: Berlin/Heidelberg, Germany, 2018; pp. 241–277. ISBN 978-3-662-55369-5.
13. Fernandes, C.; Fontaínhas-Fernandes, A.; Cabral, D.; Salgado, M.A. Heavy metals in water, sediment and tissues of liza saliens from Esmoriz–Paramos lagoon, Portugal. *Environ. Monit. Assess.* **2008**, *136*, 267–275. [CrossRef] [PubMed]
14. Magni, P.; De Falco, G.; Como, S.; Casu, D.; Floris, A.; Petrov, A.N.; Castelli, A.; Perilli, A. Distribution and ecological relevance of fine sediments in organic-enriched lagoons: The case study of the Cabras lagoon (Sardinia, Italy). *Mar. Pollut. Bull.* **2008**, *56*, 549–564. [CrossRef] [PubMed]
15. Ivanić, M.; Lojen, S.; Grozić, D.; Jurina, I.; Škapin, S.D.; Troskot-Čorbić, T.; Mikac, N.; Juračić, M.; Sondi, I. Geochemistry of sedimentary organic matter and trace elements in modern lake sediments from transitional karstic land-sea environment of the Neretva River delta (Kuti Lake, Croatia). *Quat. Int.* **2018**, *494*, 286–299. [CrossRef]
16. Froelich, P.N.; Klinkhammer, G.P.; Bender, M.L.; Luedtke, N.A.; Heath, G.R.; Cullen, D.; Dauphin, P.; Hammond, D.; Hartman, B.; Maynard, V. Early oxidation of organic matter in pelagic sediments of the eastern equatorial Atlantic: Suboxic diagenesis. *Geochim. Cosmochim. Acta* **1979**, *43*, 1075–1090. [CrossRef]
17. Rigaud, S.; Radakovitch, O.; Couture, R.-M.; Deflandre, B.; Cossa, D.; Garnier, C.; Garnier, J.-M. Mobility and fluxes of trace elements and nutrients at the sediment–water interface of a lagoon under contrasting water column oxygenation conditions. *Appl. Geochem.* **2013**, *31*, 35–51. [CrossRef]
18. Santos-Echeandía, J.; Prego, R.; Cobelo-García, A.; Caetano, M. Metal composition and fluxes of sinking particles and post-depositional transformation in a ria coastal system (NW Iberian Peninsula). *Mar. Chem.* **2012**, *134–135*, 36–46. [CrossRef]
19. Chaillou, G.; Anschutz, P.; Lavaux, G.; Schäfer, J.; Blanc, G. The distribution of Mo, U, and Cd in relation to major redox species in muddy sediments of the Bay of Biscay. *Mar. Chem.* **2002**, *80*, 41–59. [CrossRef]
20. Atkinson, C.A.; Jolley, D.F.; Simpson, S.L. Effect of overlying water pH, dissolved oxygen, salinity and sediment disturbances on metal release and sequestration from metal contaminated marine sediments. *Chemosphere* **2007**, *69*, 1428–1437. [CrossRef]
21. Morrison, S.; Nikolai, S.; Townsend, D.; Belden, J. Distribution and bioavailability of trace metals in shallow sediments from Grand Lake, Oklahoma. *Arch. Environ. Contam. Toxicol.* **2019**, *76*, 31–41. [CrossRef]
22. Natura 2000 network GR 2230001. Available online: http://filotis.itia.ntua.gr/biotopes/c/GR2230001/ (accessed on 1 August 2019).
23. Botsou, F.; Godelitsas, A.; Kaberi, H.; Mertzimekis, T.J.; Goettlicher, J.; Steininger, R.; Scoullos, M. Distribution and partitioning of major and trace elements in pyrite-bearing sediments of a Mediterranean coastal lagoon. *Chemie der Erde Geochem.* **2015**, *75*, 219–236. [CrossRef]
24. Papaspyropoulos, C. *Hydrogeological Study of Kerkyra Island*; Institute of Geology and Mineral Exploration: Athens, Greece, 1991.
25. Morfis, A.; Sfetsos, K.; Paschos, P.; Stefouli, M.; Karapanos, E.; Angelopoulos, A.; Tzoulis, C. *Study of the Diet of Groundwater Aquifer Systems of the Kerkyra Island*; Institute of Geology and Mineral Exploration: Athens, Greece, 2002.
26. Tserolas, P.; Mpotziolis, C.; Maravelis, A.; Zelilidis, A. Preliminary geochemical and sedimentological analysis in nw corfu: the miocene sediments in Agios Georgios Pagon. *Bull. Geol. Soc.* **2016**, *50*, 402–412. [CrossRef]
27. Scoullos, M.; Dassenakis, M.; Zeri, C. Trace metal behavior during summer in a stratified Mediterranean system: The Louros Estuary (Greece). *Water. Air. Soil Pollut.* **1996**, *88*, 269–295. [CrossRef]
28. Kersten, M.; Smedes, F. Normalization procedures for sediment contaminants in spatial and temporal trend monitoring. *J. Environ. Monit.* **2002**, *4*, 109–115. [CrossRef]
29. Liu, W.X.; Li, X.D.; Shen, Z.G.; Wang, D.C.; Wai, O.W.H.; Li, Y.S. Multivariate statistical study of heavy metal enrichment in sediments of the Pearl River Estuary. *Environ. Pollut.* **2003**, *121*, 377–388. [CrossRef]
30. Loring, D.H.; Rantala, R.T.T. Manual for the geochemical analyses of marine sediments and suspended particulate matter. *Earth Sci. Rev.* **1992**, *32*, 235–283. [CrossRef]
31. Grygar, T.M.; Popelka, J. Revisiting geochemical methods of distinguishing natural concentrations and pollution by risk elements in fluvial sediments. *J. Geochem. Explor.* **2016**, *170*, 39–57. [CrossRef]

32. ISO. *Soil Quality–Dissolution for the Determination of Total Element Content. Part 1: Dissolution with Hydrofluoric and Perchloric Acids*; Technical Report No. 14869-1: 2001; ISO: Geneva, Switzerland, 2001.
33. Agemian, H.; Chau, A.S.Y. Evaluation of extraction techniques for the determination of metals in aquatic sediments. *Analyst* **1976**, *101*, 761–767. [CrossRef]
34. European Commission. Directive 2000/60/EC of the European Parliament and of the Council of 23 October 2000 Establishing a Framework for Community Action in the Field of Water Policy. *Off. J. Eur. Commun.* **2000**, *L327*, 1–72.
35. European Union. Directive 2013/39/EU of the European Parliament and of the Council of 12 August 2013 Amending Directives 2000/60/EC and 2008/105/EC as Regards Priority Substances in the Field of Water Policy Text with EEA Relevance. *Off. J. Eur. Union* **2013**, *L226*, 1–17.
36. Horowitz, A.J. *A Primer on Sediment-Trace Element Chemistry*, 2nd ed.; Lewis Publishers, Inc.: Michigan, IN, USA, 1991.
37. Horowitz, A.J.; Elrick, K.A. The relation of stream sediment surface area, grain size and composition to trace element chemistry. *Appl. Geochem.* **1987**, *2*, 437–451. [CrossRef]
38. Bibby, R.L.; Webster-Brown, J.G. Characterisation of urban catchment suspended particulate matter (Auckland region, New Zealand); a comparison with non-urban SPM. *Sci. Total Environ.* **2005**, *343*, 177–197. [CrossRef] [PubMed]
39. Dassenakis, M.; Scoullos, M.; Gaitis, A. Trace metals transport and behavior in the Mediterranean estuary of Acheloos River. *Mar. Pollut. Bull.* **1997**, *34*, 103–111. [CrossRef]
40. Sholkovitz, E.R.; Boyle, E.A.; Price, N.B. The removal of dissolved humic acids and iron during estuarine mixing. *Earth Planet. Sci. Lett.* **1978**, *40*, 130–136. [CrossRef]
41. Warren, L.A.; Haack, E.A. Biogeochemical controls on metal behavior in freshwater environments. *Earth Sci. Rev.* **2001**, *54*, 261–320. [CrossRef]
42. Yuan, F.; Chaffin, J.D.; Xue, B.; Wattrus, N.; Zhu, Y.; Sun, Y. Contrasting sources and mobility of trace metals in recent sediments of western Lake Erie. *J. Great Lakes Res.* **2018**, *44*, 1026–1034. [CrossRef]
43. Warren, L.A.; Zimmermann, A.P. Suspended particulate grain size dynamics and their implications for trace metal sorption in the Don River. *Aquat. Sci.* **1994**, *56*, 348–362. [CrossRef]
44. Turner, A.; Le Roux, S.M.; Millward, G.E. Adsorption of cadmium to iron and manganese oxides during estuarine mixing. *Mar. Chem.* **2008**, *108*, 77–84. [CrossRef]
45. Charette, M.A.; Sholkovitz, E.R.; Hansel, C.M. Trace element cycling in a subterranean estuary: Part 1. Geochemistry of the permeable sediments. *Geochim. Cosmochim. Acta* **2005**, *69*, 2095–2109. [CrossRef]
46. Turner, A.; Millward, G.E.; Schuchardt, B.; Schirmer, M.; Prange, A. Trace metal distribution coefficients in the Weser Estuary (Germany). *Cont. Shelf Res.* **1992**, *12*, 1277–1292. [CrossRef]
47. Cenci, R.M.; Martin, J.-M. Concentration and fate of trace metals in Mekong River Delta. *Sci. Total Environ.* **2004**, *332*, 167–182. [CrossRef] [PubMed]
48. Cobelo-García, A.; Prego, R.; Labandeira, A. Land inputs of trace metals, major elements, particulate organic carbon and suspended solids to an industrial coastal bay of the NE Atlantic. *Water Res.* **2004**, *38*, 1753–1764. [CrossRef] [PubMed]
49. Balls, P.W. The partition of trace metals between dissolved and particulate phases in European coastal waters: A compilation of field data and comparison with laboratory studies. *Netherlands J. Sea Res.* **1989**, *23*, 7–14. [CrossRef]
50. Elbaz-Poulichet, F.; Martin, J.M.; Huang, W.W.; Zhu, J.X. Dissolved Cd behavior in some selected French and Chinese estuaries. Consequences on Cd supply to the ocean. *Mar. Chem.* **1987**, *22*, 125–136. [CrossRef]
51. Comans, R.N.J.; van Dijk, C.P.J. Role of complexation processes in cadmium mobilization during estuarine mixing. *Nature* **1988**, *336*, 151–154. [CrossRef]
52. Rozan, T.F.; Benoit, G. Geochemical factors controlling free Cu ion concentrations in river water. *Geochim. Cosmochim. Acta* **1999**, *63*, 3311–3319. [CrossRef]
53. Roussiez, V.; Ludwig, W.; Radakovitch, O.; Probst, J.-L.; Monaco, A.; Charrière, B.; Buscail, R. Fate of metals in coastal sediments of a Mediterranean flood-dominated system: An approach based on total and labile fractions. *Estuar. Coast. Shelf Sci.* **2011**, *92*, 486–495. [CrossRef]
54. Sutherland, R.A.; Tack, F.M.G.; Ziegler, A.D.; Bussen, J.O. Metal extraction from road-deposited sediments using nine partial decomposition procedures. *Appl. Geochem.* **2004**, *19*, 947–955. [CrossRef]

55. Agemian, H.; Chau, A.S.Y. A study of different analytical extraction methods for nondetrital heavy metals in aquatic sediments. *Arch. Environ. Contam. Toxicol.* **1977**, *6*, 69–82. [CrossRef]
56. Frascari, F.; Matteucci, G.; Giordano, P. Evaluation of a eutrophic coastal lagoon ecosystem from the study of bottom sediments. *Hydrobiologia* **2002**, *475*, 387–401. [CrossRef]
57. Lyle, M. The brown-green color transition in marine sediments: A marker of the Fe(III)-Fe(II) redox boundary1. *Limnol. Oceanogr.* **1983**, *28*, 1026–1033. [CrossRef]
58. Gobeil, C.; Macdonald, R.W.; Sundby, B. Diagenetic separation of cadmium and manganese in suboxic continental margin sediments. *Geochim. Cosmochim. Acta* **1997**, *61*, 4647–4654. [CrossRef]
59. Huerta-Diaz, M.A.; Morse, J.W. Pyritization of trace metals in anoxic marine sediments. *Geochim. Cosmochim. Acta* **1992**, *56*, 2681–2702. [CrossRef]
60. Berner, R.A. Sedimentary pyrite formation: An update. *Geochim. Cosmochim. Acta* **1984**, *48*, 605–615. [CrossRef]
61. Rosenthal, Y.; Lam, P.; Boyle, E.A.; Thomson, J. Authigenic cadmium enrichments in suboxic sediments: Precipitation and postdepositional mobility. *Earth Planet. Sci. Lett.* **1995**, *132*, 99–111. [CrossRef]
62. Couture, R.-M.; Hindar, A.; Rognerud, S. Emerging investigator series: Geochemistry of trace elements associated with Fe and Mn nodules in the sediment of limed boreal lakes. *Environ. Sci. Process. Impacts* **2018**, *20*, 406–414. [CrossRef] [PubMed]
63. Cooper, D.C.; Morse, J.W. Extractability of metal sulfide minerals in acidic solutions: Application to environmental studies of trace metal contamination within anoxic sediments. *Environ. Sci. Technol.* **1998**, *32*, 1076–1078. [CrossRef]
64. Birch, G.F. Determination of sediment metal background concentrations and enrichment in marine environments–A critical review. *Sci. Total Environ.* **2017**, *580*, 813–831. [CrossRef]
65. Voutsinou-Taliadouri, F. A weak acid extraction method as a tool for the metal pollution assessment in surface sediments. *Microchimica Acta* **1995**, *119*, 243–249. [CrossRef]
66. TUREKIAN, K.K.; WEDEPOHL, K.H. Distribution of the elements in some major units of the Earth's crust. *GSA Bull.* **1961**, *72*, 175–192. [CrossRef]
67. Rudnick, R.L.; Gao, S. 4.1—Composition of the continental crust. In *Treatise on Geochemistry*, 2nd ed.; Holland, H.D., Turekian, K.K., Eds.; Elsevier: Oxford, UK, 2014; pp. 1–51. ISBN 978-0-08-098300-4.
68. Tzifas, I.T.; Godelitsas, A.; Magganas, A.; Androulakaki, E.; Eleftheriou, G.; Mertzimekis, T.J.; Perraki, M. Uranium-bearing phosphatized limestones of NW Greece. *J. Geochem. Explor.* **2014**, *143*, 62–73. [CrossRef]
69. Birch, G.F.; Olmos, M.A. Sediment-bound heavy metals as indicators of human influence and biological risk in coastal water bodies. *ICES J. Mar. Sci.* **2008**, *65*, 1407–1413. [CrossRef]
70. Andrisoa, A.; Stieglitz, T.C.; Rodellas, V.; Raimbault, P. Primary production in coastal lagoons supported by groundwater discharge and porewater fluxes inferred from nitrogen and carbon isotope signatures. *Mar. Chem.* **2019**, *210*, 48–60. [CrossRef]
71. Tovar-Sánchez, A.; Basterretxea, G.; Rodellas, V.; Sánchez-Quiles, D.; García-Orellana, J.; Masqué, P.; Jordi, A.; López, J.M.; Garcia-Solsona, E. Contribution of groundwater discharge to the coastal dissolved nutrients and trace metal concentrations in Majorca Island: Karstic vs. detrital systems. *Environ. Sci. Technol.* **2014**, *48*, 11819–11827. [CrossRef] [PubMed]
72. Burnett, W.C.; Bokuniewicz, H.; Huettel, M.; Moore, W.S.; Taniguchi, M. Groundwater and pore water inputs to the coastal zone. *Biogeochemistry* **2003**, *66*, 3–33. [CrossRef]
73. Eisma, D. Flocculation and de-flocculation of suspended matter in estuaries. *Netherlands J. Sea Res.* **1986**, *20*, 183–199. [CrossRef]
74. Nolting, R.F.; Helder, W.; de Baar, H.J.W.; Gerringa, L.J.A. Contrasting behavior of trace metals in the Scheldt Estuary in 1978 compared to recent years. *J. Sea Res.* **1999**, *42*, 275–290. [CrossRef]
75. Sholkovitz, E.R. The flocculation of dissolved Fe, Mn, Al, Cu, Ni, Co and Cd during estuarine mixing. *Earth Planet. Sci. Lett.* **1978**, *41*, 77–86. [CrossRef]
76. Puig, P.; Palanques, A.; Sanchez-Cabeza, J.A.; Masqué, P. Heavy metals in particulate matter and sediments in the Southern Barcelona sedimentation system (North-Western Mediterranean). *Mar. Chem.* **1999**, *63*, 311–329. [CrossRef]

77. Karageorgis, A.P.; Gardner, W.D.; Mikkelsen, O.A.; Georgopoulos, D.; Ogston, A.S.; Assimakopoulou, G.; Krasakopoulou, E.; Oaie, G.; Secrieru, D.; Kanellopoulos, T.D.; et al. Particle sources over the Danube River delta, Black Sea based on distribution, composition and size using optics, imaging and bulk analyses. *J. Mar. Syst.* **2014**, *131*, 74–90. [CrossRef]
78. Fox, J.M.; Hill, P.S.; Milligan, T.G.; Boldrin, A. Flocculation and sedimentation on the Po River Delta. *Mar. Geol.* **2004**, *203*, 95–107. [CrossRef]

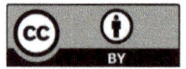

© 2019 by the authors. Licensee MDPI, Basel, Switzerland. This article is an open access article distributed under the terms and conditions of the Creative Commons Attribution (CC BY) license (http://creativecommons.org/licenses/by/4.0/).

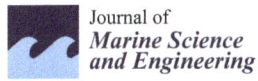

Article

Geomorphology of a Holocene Hurricane Deposit Eroded from Rhyolite Sea Cliffs on Ensenada Almeja (Baja California Sur, Mexico)

Markes E. Johnson [1,*], Rigoberto Guardado-France [2], Erlend M. Johnson [3] and Jorge Ledesma-Vázquez [2]

1   Geosciences Department, Williams College, Williamstown, MA 01267, USA
2   Facultad de Ciencias Marinas, Universidad Autónoma de Baja California,
    Ensenada 22800, Baja California, Mexico; rigoberto@uabc.edu.mx (R.G.-F.); ledesma@uabc.edu.mx (J.L.-V.)
3   Anthropology Department, Tulane University, New Orleans, LA 70018, USA; erlend.johnson@gmail.com
*   Correspondence: mjohnson@williams.edu; Tel.: +1-413-597-2329

Received: 22 May 2019; Accepted: 20 June 2019; Published: 22 June 2019

Abstract: This work advances research on the role of hurricanes in degrading the rocky coastline within Mexico's Gulf of California, most commonly formed by widespread igneous rocks. Under evaluation is a distinct coastal boulder bed (CBB) derived from banded rhyolite with boulders arrayed in a partial-ring configuration against one side of the headland on Ensenada Almeja (Clam Bay) north of Loreto. Preconditions related to the thickness of rhyolite flows and vertical fissures that intersect the flows at right angles along with the specific gravity of banded rhyolite delimit the size, shape and weight of boulders in the Almeja CBB. Mathematical formulae are applied to calculate the wave height generated by storm surge impacting the headland. The average weight of the 25 largest boulders from a transect nearest the bedrock source amounts to 1200 kg but only 30% of the sample is estimated to exceed a full metric ton in weight. The wave height calculated to move those boulders is close to 8 m. Additional localities with CBBs composed of layered rock types such as basalt and andesite are proposed for future studies within the Gulf of California. Comparisons with selected CBBs in other parts of the world are made.

Keywords: coastal boulder deposit; hurricane storm surge; hydrodynamic equations; Gulf of California (Mexico)

1. Introduction

Hurricane Odile was one of the most destructive storms to strike the Mexican state of Baja California Sur in terms of infrastructure damage [1]. It made landfall just after midnight on September 14, 2014 at Cabo San Lucas on the southern tip of the Baja California peninsula as a Category 4 hurricane packing sustained wind speeds of 144 km/h. Tracking into the Gulf of California, the maximum wind speed fell to 113 km/h by the time the storm reached the town of Loreto located 375 km to the northeast later the same day. As it advanced from under a foot-print diameter of 600 km, the system's counter-clockwise rotation spun out storm bands with the strongest winds and wind-driven waves generated from its energetic right-front quadrant. Quite aside from damage to public and private property of concern to civil authorities, erosion due to coastal flooding and the direct impact of wave activity against natural shorelines is a separate issue of interest to physical geographers and marine geologists.

Outwash from uplands through flooded stream beds has the capacity not only to transport terrestrial sediments to the coast but also to reconfigure unconsolidated shore deposits such as beaches and estuary tidal bars. Moreover, rocky shorelines are subject to incremental erosion from repeated storms and long-shore currents over time. A previous contribution from our team [2] focused on Holocene events during the last 10,000 years related to the physical erosion of rocky shores on Isla del Carmen, one of the larger fault-block islands in the gulf with 95% coverage by rocky shores. The laterally coherent coastal boulder bed (CBB) that resides 12-m above mean sea level on the east side of Isla del Carmen is distinct due its source from limestone strata vulnerable to storm waves on the outer lip of a marine terrace. Limestone accounts for only a small part of the rocky coast around that particular island, which is dominated by igneous rocks. Based on a coastal survey by Backus et al. (2009) using satellite imagery [3], igneous rocks are represented by granodiorite, andesite, basalt and other volcanic sediments to account for 34% of the shoreline in the western Gulf of California (including islands). By comparison, limestone amounts to only 7.5% of the whole.

An eye-witness account filmed during Hurricane Odile from a landmark home built into limestone cliffs north of Loreto at Ensenada Basilio recorded waves that crashed over coastal prominences at a height of 8 m above mean sea level [4]; see also Supplementary Materials. Horizontal rain reached the inner-most part of the residential compound set back from the cliff edge by some 45 m. At nearby Ensenada Almeja (Clam Bay), a north-oriented headland is formed by igneous rocks with a prominence falling from a high of 18 to 6 m above mean sea level at its distal tip. Theoretically, those cliffs are vulnerable to erosion from wave shock arriving from the east, during which winds from a tropical depression would cross from one side of the headland to the other. The object of this study is the asymmetrical boulder bed forming a semi-ring deposit exclusively on one side of the headland within Ensenada Almeja that partially restricts the bay's opening. This is the first analysis of its kind dealing with igneous rocks that form CBBs in the Gulf of California. Overall, a wide range of energy sources capable of rocky-shore erosion and CBB development include the daily tides, seasonal wind patterns that influence long-shore currents, episodic storms, and tsunamis. A secondary goal is to provide information on additional CBBs throughout the Gulf of California formed by igneous boulders. Common patterns in the physical geography of such features suggest a novel approach forward in the study of CBBs within an active zone of subtropical storms impacting continental margins. Useful comparisons also are made with notable CBBs elsewhere in the world.

2. Geographical and Geological Setting

The Gulf of California is a marginal sea between the Mexican mainland and the Baja California peninsula with a NW-SE axis 1100 km long and a 180-km wide opening to the Pacific Ocean at its southern end (Figure 1a). The sea's mean annual sea-surface temperature (SST) is 24° which is higher than the norm of 18° in the adjacent ocean and the mean average rainfall on the peninsula amounts to only 15.3 cm [5]. During relatively infrequent impact by hurricanes, conditions are dramatically altered especially in terms of heavy rainfall over desert terrain lacking thick plant cover. Tropical storms that immerge in the East Pacific Ocean typically form off the coast of Acapulco below 15° N latitude and track northward, turning outward to the west before reaching the southern tip of the Baja California peninsula at 23° N latitude. Storms that stray across the Baja California peninsula into the Gulf of California are called *chubascos*, only some of which amount to disturbances of hurricane strength. Other influences that contribute to the aggradation of coastal sediments include daily tides and seasonal winds that intermittently funnel down the axis of the gulf from the northwest with an average azimuth from N to S from December to March. This is shown by a tightly constrained rose diagram (Backus and Johnson, 2009, their figure 10.1 D), based on the orientation of structures in 84 coastal sand dunes throughout the region [6]. Strong winds capable of generating sea swells given sufficient fetch are known to blow persistently for days at a time, with gusts between 8 and 10 m/s not uncommon [7,8].

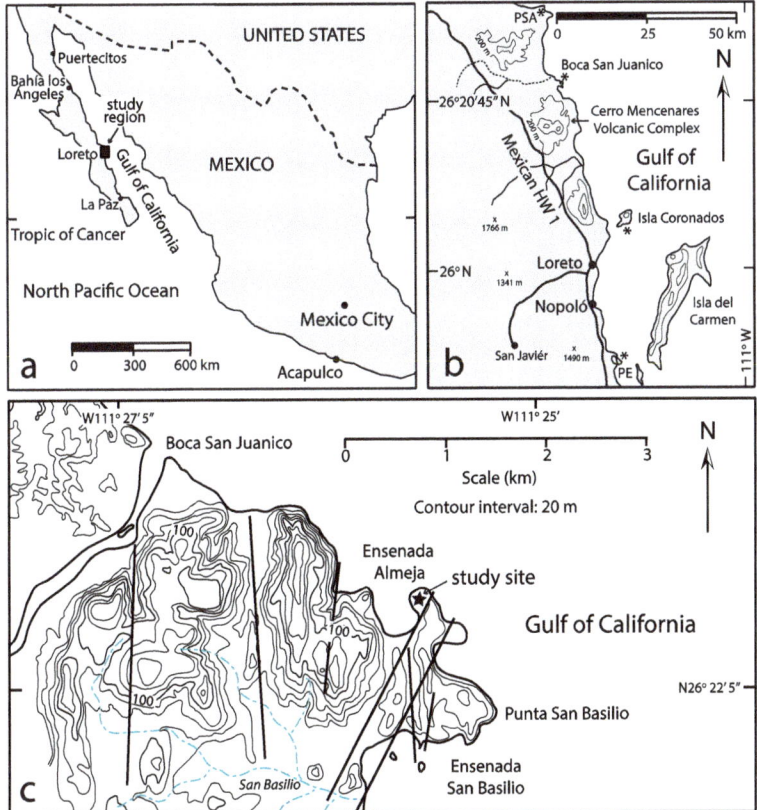

Figure 1. Locality maps showing Mexico's Baja California peninsula and Gulf of California; (**a**) Mexico and border area with the United Sates, denoting key villages or cities with dots and the study region marked by a square; (**b**) Region around Loreto in Baja California Sur, marking coastal boulder beds (*) at Puerto Escondido (PS), Isla Coronados, Ensenada Almeja near the Boca San Junico and Punta San Antonio (PSA); (**c**) Study site at Ensenada Almeja.

The geology of the San Basilio area 30 km north of Loreto (Figure 1b) incorporates the study site around Ensenada Almeja (Figure 1c), which features a landscape dominated by igneous rocks including banded rhyolite, hyaloclastite, massive rhyolite and volcanic ash [9]. Fossil-bearing limestone beds deposited around and above massive rhyolite domes are consistent with an assignment to the Zanclean Stage within the Lower Pliocene. Pleistocene deposits of consolidated dune limestone are seated above an eroded rhyolite shelf on the east side of Ensenada Almeja and extend inland through a north-south valley connected to Ensenada San Basilio. Mapping of fault lines throughout the region suggests that the low ground occupied by the Almeja CBB is separated from an adjacent rhyolite dome by a normal fault (Figure 2) parallel to a well-defined fault crossing through part of the headland to the east with a trend of N28°E to S28°W [8].

3. Materials and Methods

3.1. Data Collection

Ensenada Almeja was visited on 28 and 29 April 2019, when the original data for this study were collected based on a sample of 100 boulders divided equally among four transects crossing the CBB.

A Brunton compass and meter tape were used to lay out the transects, three of which conform to a N-S or E-W axis (Figure 2). The other transect was laid out parallel to the cliff line near the boundary fault. Various conventions exist for the differentiation of sedimentary clasts but the definition for a boulder followed in this exercise is that proposed by Wentworth (1922) for a clast equal to or greater than 256 mm in diameter [10]. No upper limit for this category is found in the geological literature, although Ruban et al. (2019) championed the term "megaclast" for boulders of extraordinary size [11]. That term is an appropriate descriptor for some of the boulders in the Almeja CBB.

The largest 25 boulders along each transect with centers spaced from 1 to 1.5 m apart were measured manually along three principle axes (long, intermediate and short). Triangular plots were employed to show variations in boulder shape, following the design of Sneed and Folk (1958) for river pebbles [12]. Data on the maximum and minimum lengths perpendicular to each other from individual boulders were fitted to bar graphs to show size variations from one transect to the next.

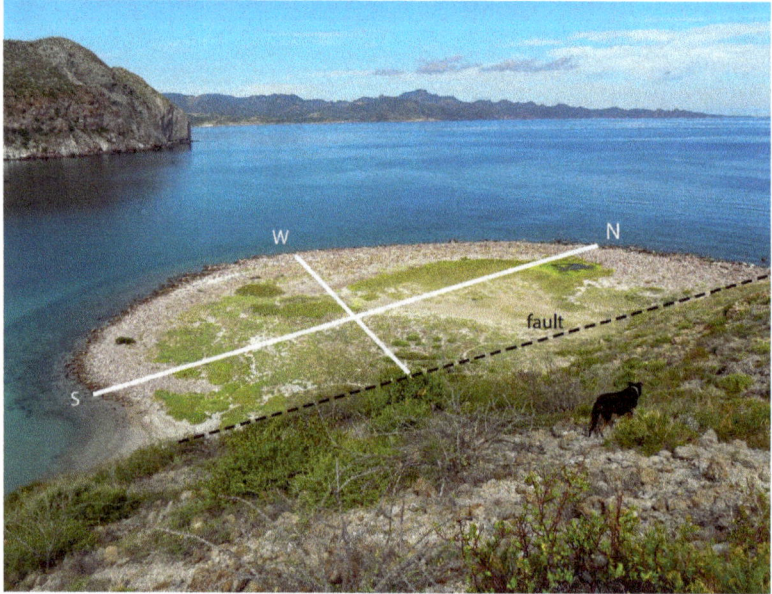

Figure 2. Northwest view across Ensenada Almeja coastal boulder bed (CBB) from an elevation of 16 m on the adjacent fault-bound headland formed by rhyolite bedrock (dog for scale on ridge).

A representative cobble of banded-rhyolite was collected from the Almeja CBB for laboratory treatment at Williams College, where it was weighed, and its volume determined as a function of equal displacement when submerged in a tank of water. Prior to immersion, the porous rhyolite sample was water-proofed by spraying it with Thompson's Water Seal ™ (The Thompson's Co., Cleveland, OH, USA).

A DJI Phantom-2 drone ™ (DJI, Nanshan District, Shenzhen, China) was flown over the Almeja headland and CBB to provide an overview of the study area and key reference points for construction of a detailed site map.

3.2. Hydraulic Model

After the weight and density of a banded-rhyolite sample is determined in the laboratory, a hydraulic model may be applied to predict the energy needed to shift larger rhyolite blocks from the headland outcrop and deposit them as a CBB in Ensenada Almeja. Along with shape, size and density, the pre-transport environment of coastal boulders factors into the wave height required for detachment and removal. Boulders derived from a weathered surface with deep joints at right angles are influenced mainly by lift force, alone. This requires somewhat higher waves to initiate transport compared to boulders already siting in a submerged position. To initiate motion of a loosened block, the lift force must overcome the force of restraint minus buoyancy, provided the block has separated completely from the basement substrate. Herein, the general formula used to calculate wave height related to CBB development is taken from the work of Nott [13], used for estimation of storm waves.

$$H_s \geq \frac{(P_s - P_w/P_w)^{2a}}{C_d(ac/b^2) + C_1}$$

where H_s = height of the storm wave at breaking point; $u = (gH)^{0.5}$ and $\partial = 1$; a, b, c = long, intermediate and short axes of the boulder (m) P_s = density of the boulder (tons/m³ or g/cm³), C_d = drag coefficient, C_m = coefficient of mass (= 2) and C_1 = lift coefficient (= 0.178);

u = instantaneous flow acceleration (= 1 m/s²)

A variation on this formula applied exclusively to joint-bounded boulders is as follows [13]:

$$H_s \geq (P_s - P_w/P_w)\, a/C_1$$

4. Results

4.1. Sample Density Calculation

The banded-rhyolite sample retrieved for laboratory analysis measures 15 × 8 × 5 cm on three axes perpendicular to one another. Due to irregularities in shape, however, it is not accurate to equate volume with a simple multiplication of the measurements in cubic centimeters (600 cm³). The weight of the sample was found to be 843.5 g. After treatment making the sample water-tight, submergence in water registered a displacement equal to 390 mL. Dividing mass by volume yielded a density of 2.16 for banded rhyolite. Checking the laboratory result for volume against the mathematical result, it was found that the actual volume is only 65% of the latter. All of the boulders in the Almeja CBB are crudely shaped with dimensions similar to a shoe box but with irregularities. Roughly the same adjustment regarding irregular shapes was taken into account when correcting for the estimated boulder weight based on the three-dimensions measured in the field.

The banded rhyolite and hyaloclastite typical of the San Basilio region are seldom found elsewhere on the Baja California peninsula, although smaller but similar rhyolite domes occur on Isla San Luis [14] to the north. The style of Pliocene volcanism at San Basilio and Quaternary volcanism at Isla San Luis are favorably compared with Quaternary rhyolites from islands in the Tyrrhenian Sea off Italy [15,16]. Although the text-book value for the specific gravity of massive rhyolite is commonly given as 2.5, values ranging between 1.6 and 2.8 were calculated for samples by Calanchi et al. (1993), from the Aeolian islands [16]. Our result for the banded rhyolite from Ensenada Almeja falls midway within that range.

4.2. Aerial Photography

An aerial photo from the drone flight on 28 April 2019 (Figure 3) shows the distinct partial-ring shape of the Almeja CBB appended against the flank of basement rocks on the west side of the headland. The boulder field does not extend into the ring's central depression. Width of the enclosing ring is greatest adjacent to the front of the headland and most narrow some 120 m back along the fault margin with basement rocks. A small patch of standing water occurs within the circular green zone close to the north inner wall of the ring.

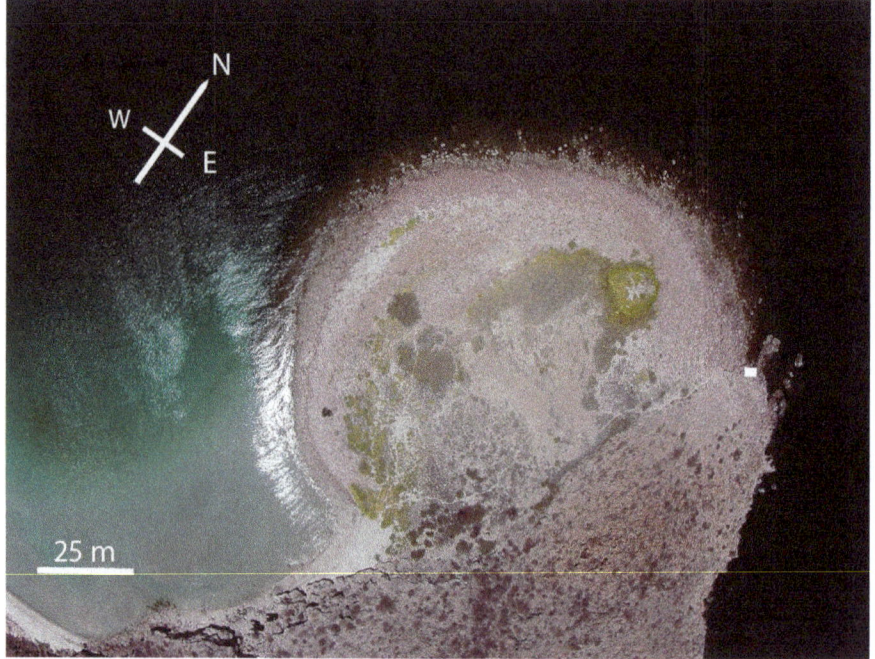

Figure 3. Aerial view directly above the Ensenada CBB showing the half-ring arrangement of the deposit on the west flank of the bedrock ridge. White rectangle on the nose of the headland marks location shown in the following field photograph (Figure 4).

4.3. Source Rock and Natural Weathering

Banded rhyolite is the dominant lithology on the headland forming the east flank of Ensenada Almeja. It is the exclusive source of eroded boulders in the Almeja CBB. The natural state of weathered bedrock is exposed in sea cliffs near the tip of the headland (Figure 3, white rectangle). From a ground view near sea level (Figure 4), the bedrock is found to be dissected by bedding planes and vertical fissures intersecting at right angles that outline oblong shapes similar to common shoe boxes. On average, such blocks are roughly three quarters of a meter in length, a half meter wide and a third of a meter in height. The apparent source of mechanical retreat worked on the rhyolite sea cliffs is hydraulic pressure exerted by wave surge against joints in the bedrock. Loosened blocks on bedding planes are poised to slide down slope into the sea aided by the force of gravity.

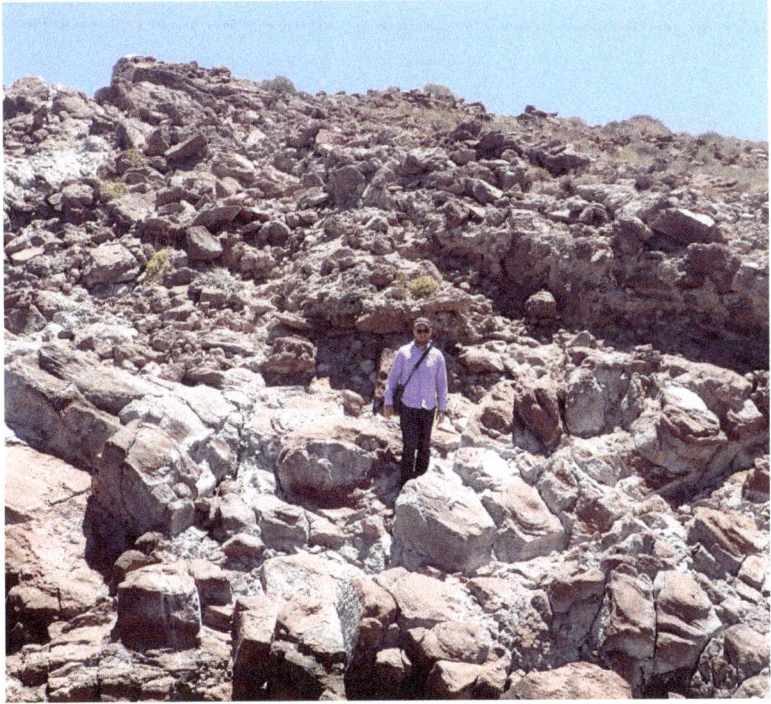

Figure 4. Bedrock exposure of banded rhyolite on the outer headland of Ensenada Almeja (see Figure 3 for location), showing pattern of intersecting vertical joints and bedding planes that facilitate boulder production under wave attack.

4.4. Mapping and Installation of Sampling Transcects

With the addition of ground measurements, the aerial photo (Figure 3) was consulted to draw a map of the Almeja CBB (Figure 5) from which different parts of the deposit could be quantified. The structure's subaerial exposure amounts to a total area of 13,000 m^2, of which the boulder field around the rim occupies close to half at 6500 m^2. As of 28 April 2019, swampy ground and open water occupied approximately 200 m^2 adjacent to the inner north wall of the ring. Bare ground covers a larger area and it is likely that over-wash of sea water enlarges the area of wet ground from time to time. The location and orientation of four transects across the CBB are marked on the map, the longest of which extends for 50 m sub-parallel to the bedrock escarpment in the northern part of the structure. The shortest is the N-S oriented transect crossing the south rim of the structure. In the central part of the Gulf of California, the maximum tidal range varies by as much as 2.75 m [17]. The subtidal portion of the Almeja CBB likely adds another 2500 m^2 to the boulder field for a total of 9000 m^2.

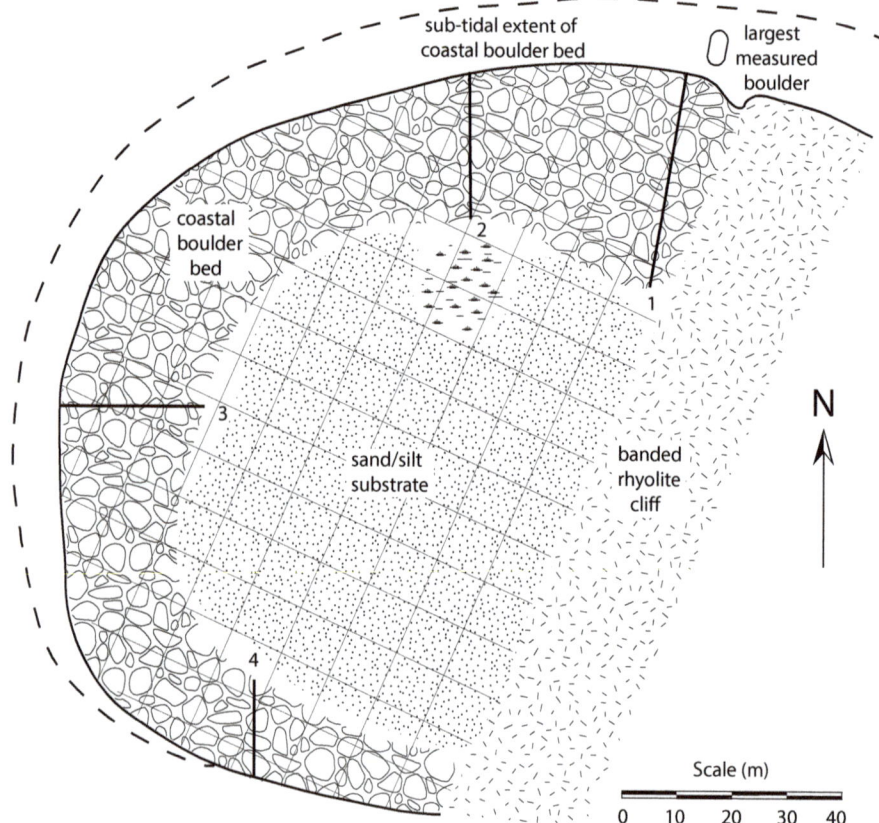

Figure 5. Map of the Ensenada Almeja CBB with location of four transects used to collect data on boulder size and shape. Each square on the superimposed grid represents 100 square meters.

The tape measure laid out along transect 1 is shown in place (Figure 6a), with a mega-boulder adjacent to the first author. It turned out to be the second largest individual boulder measured in the Almeja CBB, with a long axis of 268 cm and an estimated volume of 2000 cubic decimeters. The weight of the boulder is estimated conservatively to be on the order of 3450 kg. The height of the boulder ring above the swampy ground on transect 2 stands at 1.85 m (Figure 6b). At its farthest extent seaward to the north, the base of large boulders sits in water up to 2 m below mean sea level. The largest rhyolite boulder encountered during offshore exploration from the northeast corner of the Almeja CBB is estimated to measure 6 m in length by 3 m wide and 2 m high (Figure 5).

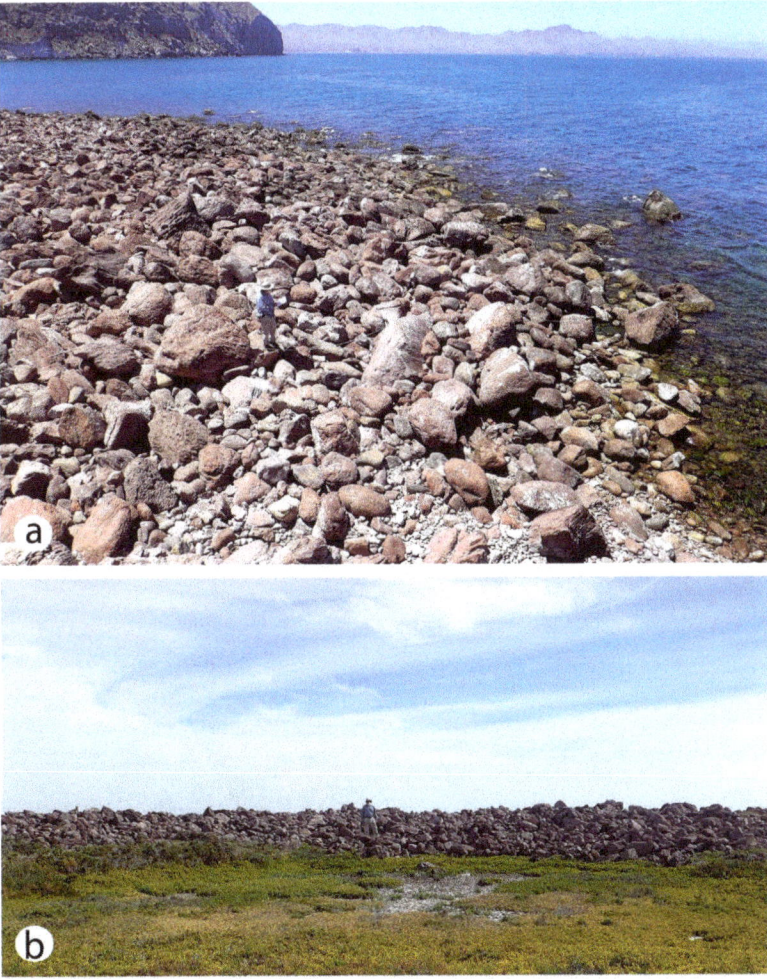

Figure 6. Northern part of the Almeja CBB; (**a**) View to the northwest across Ensenada Almeja crossing the path of Transect 1 (see Figure 5)—the largest boulders in the deposit belong to this sector (figure for scale); (**b**) View due north, showing the deposit's inner wall diagonal to Transect 2 (figure for scale).

4.5. Analysis of Boulder Shapes

Raw data on boulder size in three dimensions collected from each of four transects across the Almeja CBB are available in Appendix A (Tables A1–A4). Points representing individual blocks grouped by transect are plotted on a set of Sneed-Folk triangular diagrams (Figure 7a–d), showing the actual variation in shapes.

Those points clustered closest to the center of the diagram are most faithful to an intermediate value. With only rare occurrences registered, the absence of points at the top of the triangle signifies that no boulders eroded from equidimensional cubes are present in the sample. Also, the lack of points in the lower, left tier of the triangle demonstrates that squarely plate-shaped blocks are completely absent from the assemblies. Overall, the points grouped from different transects trace similar trends in direction from the center to the lower right tier of the diagram. The recurrent relationship denotes the presence of subpopulations of elongated boulders in the shape of shoe boxes. The significance of such diagrams puts a heavy emphasis on the thickness of parent rhyolite flows and the spacing of intersecting vertical joints in the bedrock (Figure 4). This result has a direct bearing on the relative ease with which individual blocks might be pried loose from the bedrock by wave action and fall into the sea. The process of rounding is expected to occur from the grinding of blocks against one another under wave surge against the headland. Although the trends in shape are similar among the samples from different transects (Figure 7), the plots have no bearing on variations in boulder size.

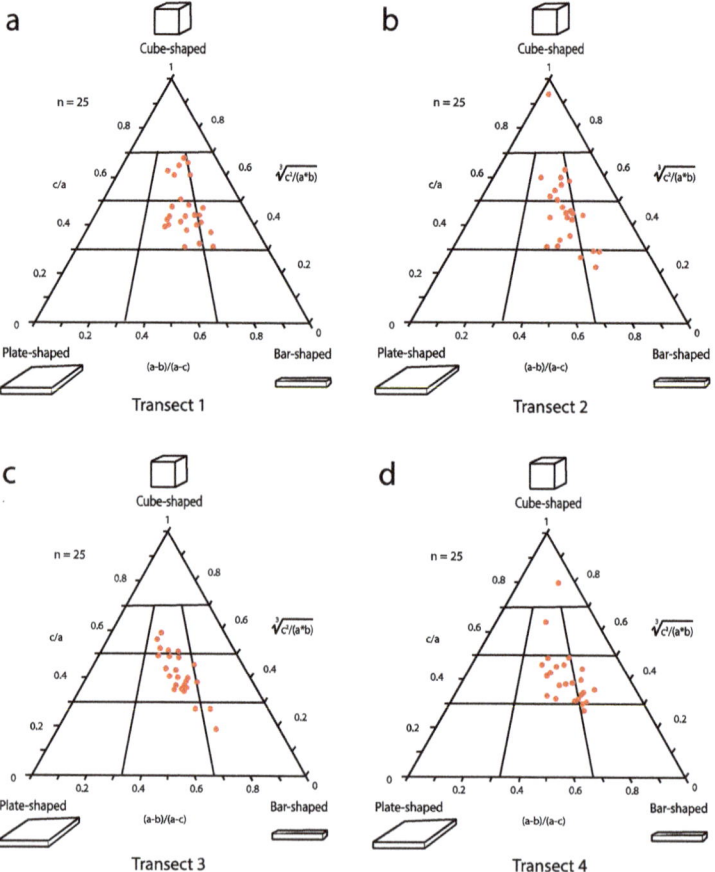

Figure 7. Set of triangular Sneed-Folk diagrams used to appraise variations in boulder shape; (**a**) Trend for boulders from Transect 1; (**b**) Trend for boulders from Transect 2; (**c**) Trend for boulders from Transect 3; (**d**) Trend for boulders from Transect 4. Note: All trends slope to the lower right, indicating shapes conserved by elongated boulders.

4.6. Analysis of Boulder Sizes

Variations in boulder size as a function of maximum and minimum length drawn from the data sets (Tables A1–A4) may be plotted separately for each transect using bar graphs. Groupings separated by intervals of 25 cm are plotted in histograms stacked to show the trend in diminishing boulder size as a function of distance from the headland source (Figure 8). The largest boulders in the Almeja CBB occur in Transect 1, the distal end of which is 12 m from the closest rhyolite sea cliff (Figure 5). The range in maximum boulder length in Transect 1 is from 58 to 268 cm (Table A1) but the highest frequency falls within the interval of 101 to 125 cm (Figure 8a). The distal end of Transect 2 meets sea level at a distance of 52 m west along the curve from the bedrock source (Figure 5). The range in maximum boulder length from Transect 2 is from 62 to 172 cm (Table A2) but the largest blocks fall into an interval a full meter less in size than the largest class in Transect 1 (Figure 8b).

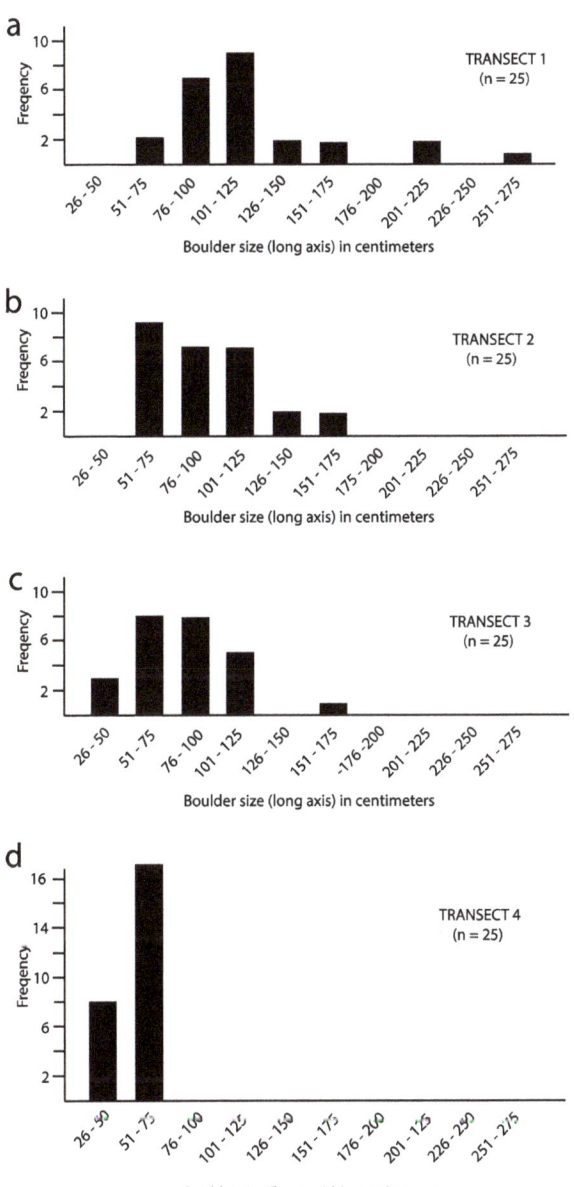

Figure 8. Set of bar graphs used to appraise variations in maximum boulder length; (**a**) Size-range and frequency for boulders from Transect 1; (**b**) Same graphic coverage for Transect 2; (**c**) Same graphic coverage for Transect 3; (**d**) Same graphic coverage for Transect 4.

The distal end of Transect 3 joins sea level on the west side of the Almeja CBB, located approximately 160 m down shore from the bedrock source through a curve (Figure 5). The range in maximum boulder length recorded from Transect 3 is from 38 to 164 cm (Table A3) but the largest two populations fall equally into neighboring classes from 51 to 100 cm (Figure 8c). For the most part, boulder populations in transects 2 and 3 overlap in range but the latter includes a smaller population rejected from among the largest 25 samples in all other transects. In contrast, the distal end of Transect 4 intersects sea level on the south margin of the Almeja CBB. At that location, the shore is approximately 230 m along the curve from the same source rocks supplying boulders to the other transect populations (Figure 5). The range in maximum boulder length from Transect 4 is from 33 to 75 cm (Table A4) but by far the largest population occurs within the interval from 51 to 75 cm (Figure 8d).

A similar trend is shown by bar graphs representing minimum boulder length recorded in Tables A1–A4. The range in minimum boulder length from transects 1 and 2 (Figure 9a,b) is significantly greater than found in transects 3 and 4 (Figure 9c,d). By far, the largest populations in transects 1–3 occur in the interval of 26 to 50 cm, although many more clasts in the interval with a maximum size of 25 cm were recorded in Transect 4 (Figure 9d). Clasts with this minimum size are abundant throughout the entire Almeja CBB but were not among the largest 25 samples recorded for minimum length in Transect 1.

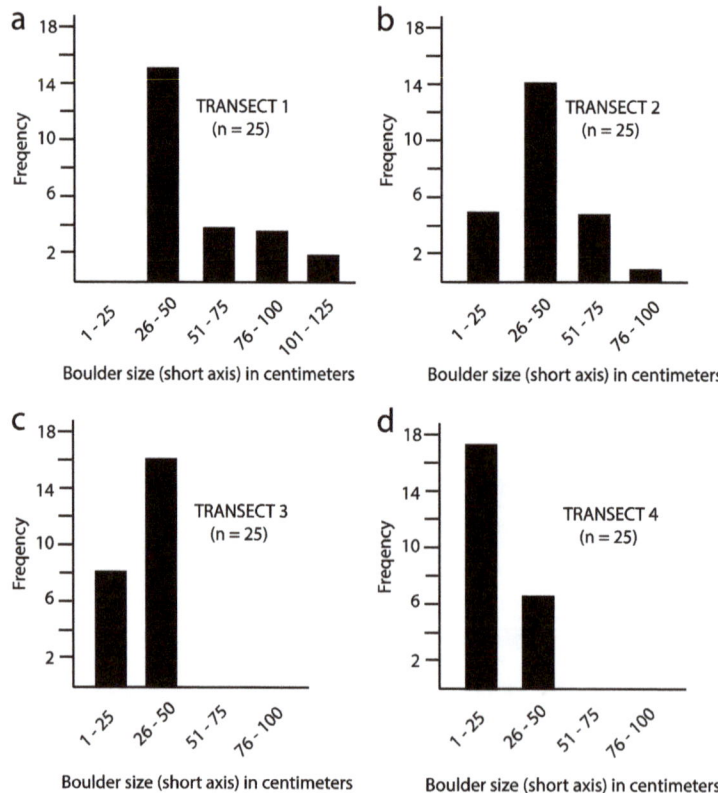

Figure 9. Set of bar graphs used to appraise variations in minimum boulder length; (**a**) Size-range and frequency for boulders from Transect 1; Transect 2 (**b**); Transect 3 (**c**); Transect 4 (**d**).

4.7. Estimation of Wave Heights

A summary of key data is provided (Table 1), pertaining to average boulder size and maximum boulder size from transects 1 to 4 as correlated with weight calculated on the basis of specific gravity for banded rhyolite. These data are employed to estimate the wave heights required to transport boulders from the bedrock source in sea cliffs to their place in the Almeja CBB. The estimated wave height needed to move the largest boulder encountered in Transect 1 amounts to 13.7 m but that for the largest boulder from Transect 4 is much less at 4.7 m. Estimates using the same equations based on the hydraulic model presented in Section 3.2 are applied to the average boulder weights from Table 1, showing a steady decrease in estimated wave heights from Transect 1 in the most exposed location to Transect 4 in the most sheltered location well within Ensenada Almeja.

Although many of the largest boulders from each transect occur closer to the outer margin and often stand at mean sea level, there are many others that sit well within the CBB. Especially in the western and southern parts of the Almeja CBB, two distinct topographic levels are present. Quantitatively, however, there is no difference in boulder shapes between the inner and outer parts of the deposit. Significantly, the estimated average wave height from the most exposed part of the Almeja CBB on Transect 1 is in agreement with direct observations of wave surge on the rocky shores on the nearby Ensenada San Basilio.

Table 1. Summary data from Appendix A (Tables A1–A4) showing maximum boulder size and estimated weight compared to the average values for all boulders (N = 25) from each of transects 1–4 together with calculated values for wave heights estimated as necessary for CBB mobility.

Tran-Sect	Number of Samples	Average Boulder Size (cm^3)	Average Boulder Weight (kg)	Estimated Average Wave ht. (m)	Max. Boulder Size (cm^3)	Max. Boulder Weight (kg)	Estimated Wave Height (m)
1	25	549,340	1,201	7.9	2,264,933	4892	13.7
2	25	182,974	395	6.0	608,546	1314	8.5
3	25	111,118	240	5.3	495,050	1069	10.3
4	25	34,032	69	3.5	111,004	240	4.7

5. Discussion

5.1. Tidal Influence on Coastal Sediment Production

The most extreme tidal range in the Gulf of California is located in the far north around the delta of the Colorado River, where a macrotidal regime with maximum amplitudes of 12 m plays out over a very low regional slope that results in tidal flats stretching seaward by more than 2 km at low tide [18]. High wave height achieved under wave surge during a major storm that coincides in timing with a high tide can be expected to influence the placement of marine sediments at a higher elevation in any given storm deposit. In the upper gulf region, those sediments are dominated by a peculiar species of marine bivalve (*Mulinia coloradoensis*), the disarticulated shells of which form major intertidal banks called *cheniers* [18]. Tides of this magnitude are unique to the upper part of the gulf. Normally, the daily shift in tidal action during calm weather should have little effect on a particular CBB in the central part of the Gulf of California, where the Guaymas Basin is quite deep. In the case of Ensenada Almeja, the daily tidal cycle does influence the sand beach at the south end of the bay. The modern beach and inland dunes that encroach on the fault valley connected to Ensenada San Basilio [9] are dominated by carbonate sand derived from the abundant bivalve mollusks giving the place its name: Clam Bay. Infaunal bivalves that burrow into the bay's sandy bottom are sheltered during low tide but the disarticulated shells of expired bivalves are liable to be uncovered by currents that accompany changes in the tidal cycle. North-facing sandy beaches in other parts of the central gulf region are commonly enriched by carbonate sand resulting from the breakdown of the abundant bivalve mollusks most commonly belonging to the species *Megapitaria squalida* [8,17].

5.2. Seasonal Wind Patterns and Long-Shore Currents

Stiff winds affecting the Gulf of California on an annual basis from November to May [5,7] are capable of generating large-scale wave trains that build in size and travel south over a wide fetch of open water. When sea swells cross into shallow water on approach to a north-facing shoreline, larger waves and surf may be generated that contribute to the abrasion of rocky shores. This action adds finer sediments to local beaches, often enriched by the abrasion of mollusk shells (see above). Such wave activity commonly occurs under clear skies in full sunshine that cannot otherwise be construed as stormy weather. Based on personal boating experience (MEJ), south-directed sea swells with an amplitude of 2 m and wavelength of approximately 10 m are not unusual along the coast near the study site during a wind event lasting several days. In the case of Ensenada Almeja, the waves originating from this source will impact the adjoining, north-facing rocky headland. Some amount of erosion can be expected against the exposed bedrock. However, this particular energy source does not account for the strikingly asymmetrical configuration of the Ensenada Almeja CBB. As apparent from aerial surveillance (Figure 3), the amount of boulder debris eroded from the east side of the headland is insignificant compared to the partial-ring CBB accumulated on the west side. Long-shore currents generated by the seasonal north winds in the region are insufficient to account for the geomorphology of the Almeja CBB.

5.3. Extra-regional Tsunami Activity

Deposits correlated with extreme wave action in other parts of the Mexico's Pacific coastline have raised the question as to whether a source from tsunamis can be distinguished from major storms [19]. In particular, the adjoining Jalisco and Michoacán states of Mexico far south of Baja California Sur are bordered by an active subduction zone resulting from compression between the Rivera lithospheric plate and the continental mainland. Among the historical events recorded for this region, the 22 June 1932 earthquake (magnitude 7.7) was one of the region's most destructive affecting an area 1 km inland along a 20-km stretch of coast with a run-up of 15 m [20]. In contrast, the Gulf of California has no historical record of tsunami events, although shallow earthquakes are relatively common due to transtensional tectonics associated with activity along multiple strike-slip faults that dissect narrow sea-floor spreading zones [5]. Traces of former subduction zones related to the San Benito and Tosco-Abreojos faults extend offshore along much of the outer Pacific coast of Baja California but these ceased to be active approximately 12 million years ago [5]. Rocky shores along the inner gulf coast of the Baja California peninsula close to the study site entail steep cliffs that rise abruptly to elevations as high as 100 m (Figure 1c). Nothing has been described as remotely similar to the Pleistocene tsunami deposits documented with a run-up of 270 m against the steep volcanic shores of Santiago in the Cape Verde Islands [21]. The hypothesis of a tsunami origin for the Ensenada Almeja CBB is easily eliminated on account of the barren zone lacking boulders inside the partial-ring construction (Figure 5), as well as the occurrence of the CBB restricted to one side of Ensenada Almeja. Any potential tsunami source would have filled the interior of the half-ring with boulders. Moreover, comparable deposits can be expected to have formed along both sides of the bay.

5.4. Hurricane Frequency

As many as 25 to 30 tropical depressions originate each year near Acapulco off western Mexico between the months of May and November before intensifying in strength and shifting northwest into the eastern Pacific Ocean [22]. Especially during El Niño events every 6 to 8 years, a few storms turn northward into the Gulf of California. In recent years, several hurricanes have struck the southern tip of the Baja California peninsula and followed tracks crossing Isla Cerralvo in the southern gulf region, where heavy rainfall flushes arroyo sediments to form tide-water deltas at some 39 localities around the island's circumference [23]. Long-shore currents stimulated by the winter winds also play a role in truncating those deltas and sending the sediment load south along both sides of the island. Hurricanes that manage to enter the gulf usually lose energy rapidly before continuing as downgraded storms, although Hurricane Odile is a recent exception, reaching Loreto at hurricane strength in 2014. The driest part of the Baja California peninsula is located far to the north in the upper Gulf of California, where normal rainfall amounts to only 5 cm per year. A remnant of Hurricane Odile was the last big storm to bring excess water to the area. In particular, the large Costilla Delta that empties sediments from Heme Canyon south of Puertecitos (Figure 1a) lends evidence to the effect of episodic rain storms that flush the region, although a nearby salt lagoon also attests to long periods of aridity [24]. The bar that closes off the salt lagoon was constructed under the influence of long-shore currents based on the occurrence of pumice cobbles derived from strata within Heme Canyon and transferred seaward via the Costilla Delta.

Although clearly episodic in frequency and less common in the northern Gulf of California, hurricanes are the major factor capable of expending sufficient energy to shape the landscapes of peninsular Baja California through the agencies of stream erosion and shore modification. The Almeja CBB, in particular, stands out as a prime example of a large but distinctly asymmetrical deposit that only could have been formed under the influence of incremental additions due to Holocene hurricanes with a counter-clockwise rotation sending wave surge westward across the headland.

5.5. Human Occupation of the San Basilio Area

Archeological evidence of kitchen middens including worked flakes of obsidian occurs on the northwest shore of Ensenada San Basilio in one of the most sheltered corners of the bay. Cave paintings also are known from a locality on the south side of the bay. These remains indicate that the area has a history of occupation predating the arrival of Europeans. No trace of habitation is known from nearby Ensenada Almeja, possibly because of exposure to the seasonal north winds. Nonetheless, native peoples would have been subjected to storm conditions from time to time.

5.6. Regional Patterns for Coastal Boulder Beds

Study of rocky-shore attrition around the Gulf of California due to impact by hurricanes through the last 10,000 years has barely commenced with the only previous example based on the limestone CBB on the east coast of Isla del Carmen [2]. The largest up-turned blocks of layered limestone from the Carmen CBB are estimated to weigh between 5.8 and 28 metric tons. The largest megaclast in the Almeja CBB (Table A1, Transect 1) is close to 5 metric tons in weight. Approximately 30% of the megaclasts measured from Transect 1 exceed one metric ton in weight. By comparison, only two of the megaclasts from the next transect (Table A2, Transect 2) exceed one metric ton in weight and only one from the third transect (Table A3) exceeds that amount. None of the boulders in the last transect (Table A4) come close to a metric ton.

To what extent might other examples of Holocene or older Pleistocene CBBs exist throughout the Gulf of California and what source rocks are most typically represented? The Loreto area offers additional possibilities for expanded studies. Located 23 km south of Loreto (Figure 1b), Puerto Escondido is a natural harbor with a single entrance from the southeast leading to a large inner lagoon sheltered by islets linked by boulder barriers eroded from an adjacent headland (El Chino) at one end and the largest island (La Enfermeria) at the other. Overall, the andesite clasts on the barriers are poorly sorted with a wide range of sizes similar to the Almeja CBB. Future research may determine to what extent the barriers were formed by long-shore currents or a combination of factors including storm activity.

A short distance north of Loreto, the south shore of Isla Coronados (Figure 1b) is clad by andesite boulders forming an extensive berm. Given that the south shore is on the leeward side of the island sheltered from the north winds and related sea swell, the berm is more likely to have been activated by hurricane activity. In addition, a Pleistocene lagoon inland from the unconsolidated boulder berm is filled with limestone that dips northward away from a bedrock ridge with the internal carbonate layers interpreted as over-wash deposits derived from rhodolith debris [25]. The most likely mechanism for north-directed over-wash events on Isla Coronados would have resulted from major storms or hurricanes arriving from the south.

A fitting analog for the Almeja CBB is the 400-m long paleoshore near Punta San Antonio (Figure 1b), formed by mixed granodiorite and andesite boulders to which a diverse Pleistocene biota is attached in growth position [26]. In particular, granodiorite boulders derive from the adjacent headland at Punta San Antonio that occupies a flanking position comparable to the rhyolite headland at Ensenada Almeja. The paleogeography of the Punta San Antonio site also features a former embayment comparable in size to Ensenada Almeja. As there is no bedrock exposure of granodiorite north of the former bay, wind-driven currents from that direction could not have been responsible for development of the Pleistocene CBB. The only alternative is an energy source associated with the passage of Pleistocene hurricanes with a counter-clockwise rotation suited to erosion of the Punta San Antonio headland to the east.

Another area with rich potential for future studies on CBBs is located in the upper Gulf of California off Bahía Los Angeles (Figure 1a). The southeast end of Isla Angel de la Guarda is known for its closed lagoons with elevated salinities that favor living microbial colonies [27], commonly recognized by paleontologists and geologists as stromatolites. Based on personal exploration (MEJ and JL-V), the smaller lagoon on Isla Angel de la Guarda (Figure 10, number 1) is closed off by a CBB formed by large andesite boulders. The principal source for this material is the adjacent rocky shore to the north, which features eroded sea stacks. As long-shore currents from the north are blocked by nearby Isla Estanque, the alternative energy source for erosion of the andesite cliffs close to the small lagoon is likely to have been the result of episodic storms or hurricanes. Based again on personal experience, andesite clasts on the deposit closing off the larger lagoon on Angel de la Guarda (Figure 10, number 2) are mostly the size of cobbles. Long-shore drift may have been more constructive in the development of the enclosing berm. Isla Estanque has yet to be explored with any focus on lagoon development (Figure 10, numbers 3 and 4) but the clock-wise rotation of storm systems offers a promising hypothesis for the development of boulder spurs yet to completely isolate related lagoons.

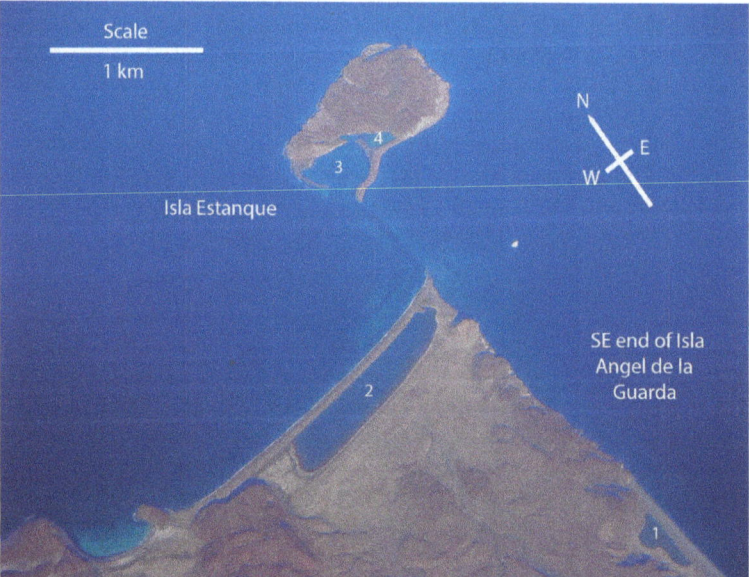

Figure 10. Aerial photo from an altitude of 15,000 m showing boulder deposits from the southeast coast of Isla Angel de la Guarda in the upper Gulf of California that define closed lagoons (1 and 2) and distinct spurs formed by bolder deposits on Isla Estanque in the process of closing other lagoons (3 and 4).

5.7. Comparison to Selected CBBs Elsewhere in the World

Ruban et al. (2019) compiled a representative collection of 58 published studies concerning Earth-bound processes capable of producing megaclasts [11]. From this sample, more than half (53%) are limited to boulder deposits that formed during Quaternary time, 20 of which represent coastal depositional settings. The data base distinguishes between Quaternary CBBs attributed to storms as opposed to tsunamis in nearly equal parts. A clear-cut example of a huge tsunami event derives from the study by Ramalho et al. (2015) with regard to basalt megaclasts as much as 8 m in diameter with a maximum estimated weight of as much as 1000 metric tons, left high on the flanks of Santiago in the Cape Verde Islands [21]. An equally clear-cut study by Cox et al. (2018) relates to blocks with an estimated weight as much as 620 metric tons pealed back from Carboniferous limestone layers exposed at the top of high sea cliffs in western Ireland [28] that are unequivocally linked to major sea storms. Not included in the data base of Ruban et al. (2019) are other studies on massive carbonate megaclasts from the Bahamas and Bermuda interpreted ambiguously as either tsunami or storm-related [29] or unequivocally as storm related [30]. Current literature on Quaternary CBBs appears to be skewed towards studies on carbonate megaclasts, such as the work by Biolchi et al. (2019) from the northern Adriatic Sea [31]. Bedded limestone formations exposed in sea cliffs are especially vulnerable to erosion by storm-induced waves, as exemplified by our previous study on a Holocene CBB from Isla del Carmen in the Gulf of California [2]. Volcanic flows composed of layered basalt and andesite also form extensive sea cliffs around the Gulf of California [3] and many other parts of the world. The geomorphology of CBBs stripped from igneous basement rocks is underrepresented in the literature and offers a research target worthy of future investigations especially in the context of likely hurricane deposits.

6. Conclusions

- Hurricanes strike Mexico's Baja California peninsula and enter the Gulf of California with increased frequency especially during El Niño years commonly repeated every 6 to 8 years. The last hurricane known to reach Ensenada Almeja in the San Basilio area north of Loreto was Hurricane Odile in 2014.
- By process of elimination taking into account more frequent but less energetic sources of input such as tidal forces, seasonal wind patterns involved with long-shore currents, as well as tsunamis, data are found to favor an incremental accumulation of the Ensenada Almeja CBB due to a repetition of hurricane events through Holocene time.
- Maximum wave height stimulated by a major storm necessary to erode the largest blocks of banded rhyolite with a calculated specific gravity of 2.16 is estimated to have been on the order of 13.7 m.
- Evidence based on size distribution in boulders from four different transects crossing perpendicular through the Almeja CBB shows a decrease in maximum size along a curved shoreline ending 230 m distal from the bedrock source on the outer tip of the adjacent headland. Loss of energy is due to wave refraction entering Ensenada Almeja after impact against the headland with wave surge arriving from the east driven by a counter-clockwise rotation of a hurricane system.
- The restriction of embayments by CBBs and the related closure of lagoons by boulder spurs in the form of unconsolidated bars, derived from bedrock sources of basalt and andesite, is a widespread pattern in the Gulf of California. Future efforts that distinguish between different energy sources related to coastal erosion of exposed bedrock must take into consideration the importance of hurricanes and down-graded tropical storms that impact the region on an episodic basis. Like rhyolite (this study), basalt and andesite are susceptible to intense hydrologic pressure exerted against parting seams and vertical joints exposed to wave action during major storms.

Supplementary Materials: The following video is available online at http://www.mdpi.com/2077-1312/7/6/193/s1, Video Hurricane Odile at San Basilio.mov.

Author Contributions: Initial field reconnaissance was conducted by M.E.J. and J.L.-V. in March 2017 with a follow-up visit by J.L.-V. in March 2018 paying close attention to patterns of natural weathering in the rhyolitic basement rocks exposed on the headland at Ensenada Almeja. Fieldwork resulting in collection of shape and size data at the Almeja CBB was carried out in May 2019 by M.E.J. and E.M.J. M.E.J. prepared the first draft of this contribution, drafted all figures and supplied all ground photos. R.G.-F. was responsible for working out the mathematics related to storm hydrodynamics.

Funding: This research received no external funding.

Acknowledgments: Foremost, we are indebted to Norm Christy, part-time resident of Loreto, for his invaluable assistance with logistics during our 2019 visit and for launching his DJI Phantom-2 drone to provide aerial photos of the Ensenada Almeja CBB. Eric Stevens provided critical insight with his video of storm action at San Basilio during Hurricane Odile. Special thanks are due to Tom Woodard in Loreto for arranging our stay at the Spanish Contessa's house at the conclusion of the project. M.E.J. is grateful to Jay Racela (Environmental Lab, Williams College) for help with the experimental calculation of density for the banded rhyolite sample from Ensenada Almeja. Reviews of an earlier manuscript for which the authors are most grateful were provided by two anonymous readers, as well as by Dmitry A. Ruban (Geology and Geography Faculty, Southern Federal University, Russia).

Conflicts of Interest: The authors declare no conflict of interest.

Appendix A

Table A1. Quantification of boulder size, volume and estimated weight from CBB samples through Transect 1 at Ensenada Almeja. The laboratory result for density of banded rhyolite at 2.16 gm/cm^3 is applied uniformly to all samples in this table.

Sample	Distance to Next (cm)	Long Axis (cm)	Intermediate Axis (cm)	Short Axis (cm)	Volume (cm^3)	Adjust. to 65%	Weight (kg)	Estimated Wave ht. (m)
1	0	88	44	38	147,136	95,638	207	5.5
2	+20	58	40	36	83,520	54,288	219	3.6
3	+60	108	60	44	285,120	185,328	296	6.8
4	+90	70	64	47	210,560	136,864	647	4.4
5	+104	110	81	523	463,320	301,158	651	6.9
6	+320	116	74	50	429,200	278,980	603	7.3
7	+108	112	82	45	413,280	268,632	580	7.0
8	+100	92	52	43	205,712	133,713	289	5.8
9	+100	155	115	93	1,657,725	1,077,521	2327	9.7
10	+140	92	88	60	485,760	315,744	682	5.8
11	+208	208	118	78	2,470,624	1,605,906	3469	13.0
12	+330	120	56	50	336,000	218,400	472	7.5
13	+220	268	111	104	3,093,792	2,010,965	4344	16.8
14	+150	97	74	30	215,340	139,971	302	6.1
15	+100	153	126	98	1,889,244	1,228,009	2653	9.6
16	+150	108	84	44	399,168	259,459	560	6.8
17	+80	105	60	33	207,900	135,135	292	6.6
18	+0	92	80	34	250,240	162,656	351	5.8
19	+120	125	118	75	1,106,250	719,063	1553	7.8
20	+0	87	66	38	218,196	141,827	306	5.5
21	+100	130	121	60	943,800	613,470	1325	8.2
22	+200	214	94	85	1,709,860	1,111,409	2401	13.4
23	+0	78	62	334	164,424	106,876	231	4.9
24	+100	128	53	38	257,792	167,565	362	8.0
25	+100	218	148	108	3,484,512	2,264,933	4892	13.7
Average	+158	125	83	57	845,139	549,340	1201	7.9

Table A2. Quantification of boulder size, volume and estimated weight from CBB samples through Transect 2 at Ensenada Almeja. The laboratory result for density of banded rhyolite at 2.16 gm/cm^3 is applied uniformly to all samples in this table.

Sample	Distance to Next (cm)	Long Axis (cm)	Intermediate Axis (cm)	Short Axis (cm)	Volume (cm^3)	Adjust. to 65%	Weight (kg)	Estimated Wave ht. (m)
1	0	83	63	24	125,496	81,572	176	5.2
2	+130	62	31	60	30,752	19,989	43	3.9
3	+220	74	45	33	49,728	32,323	70	4.6
4	+200	66	50	34	98,010	63,707	138	4.1
5	+600	172	67	46	122,400	79,560	172	10.8
6	+140	86	69	21	284,832	185,141	400	5.4
7	+260	68	27	26	38,556	25,061	54	4.3
8	+150	75	35	25	65,626	42,656	92	4.7
9	+700	64	48	29	89,089	57,907	125	4.0
10	+150	128	42	39	209,664	136,282	294	8.0
11	+130	61	56	38	129,808	84,375	182	3.8
12	+900	98	81	28	222,264	144,472	312	6.2
13	+200	92	58	55	293,480	190,762	412	5.8
14	+0	74	51	33	124,542	80,952	175	4.6
15	+800	108	64	38	262,656	170,726	369	6.8
16	+310	115	83	48	458,160	297,804	643	7.2
17	+10	125	85	53	563,125	336,031	726	7.8
18	+200	108	85	48	440,640	286,416	619	6.8
19	+100	106	55	45	262,350	170,528	368	6.7
20	+220	113	71	58	465,334	302,467	653	7.1
21	0	135	95	73	936,225	608,546	1314	8.5
22	+330	83	78	48	310,752	201,993	436	5.2
23	+250	88	73	88	234,048	217,131	469	5.5
24	+40	94	91	19	752,752	489,293	1057	5.9
25	+60	101	93	44	413,292	268,640	583	6.3
Average		100	91	63	41	283,343	182,974	395	6.0

Table A3. Quantification of boulder size, volume and estimated weight from CBB samples through Transect 3 at Ensenada Almeja. The laboratory result for density of banded rhyolite at 2.16 gm/cm^3 is applied uniformly to all samples in this table.

Sample	Distance to next (cm)	Long axis (cm)	Intermediate axis (cm)	Short axis (cm)	Volume (cm^3)	Adjust. to 65%	Weight (kg)	Estimated Wave ht. (m)
1	0	79	38	21	63,042	40,977	89	5.0
2	+400	76	53	38	153,064	99,492	215	4.8
3	+100	64	34	22	47,872	31,117	67	4.0
4	+260	54	32	23	39,744	25,834	56	3.4
5	+200	72	40	26	74,880	48,672	105	4.5
6	0	45	37	20	33,300	21,645	47	2.8
7	+120	38	25	15	14,250	9263	20	2.4
8	+800	65	36	23	53,820	34,983	76	4.1
9	+270	46	25	18	20,700	13,455	29	2.9
10	+230	109	53	20	115,510	75,101	162	6.8
11	+800	111	56	48	298,363	193,939	419	7.0
12	+130	100	50	48	240,000	156,000	337	6.3
13	+220	66	37	34	83,028	53,968	117	4.1
14	+230	75	36	27	72,900	47,385	102	4.7
15	+40	69	40	38	104,880	68,178	147	4.3
16	+20	89	55	45	220,275	143,179	309	5.6
17	+170	99	43	34	144,738	94,080	203	6.2
18	+240	76	48	44	160,512	104,333	225	4.8

Table A3. Cont.

Sample	Distance to next (cm)	Long axis (cm)	Intermediate axis (cm)	Short axis (cm)	Volume (cm³)	Adjust. to 65%	Weight (kg)	Estimated Wave ht. (m)
19	+120	75	56	28	117,600	76,440	165	4.7
20	+60	83	50	40	166,000	107,900	233	5.2
21	+220	120	58	48	334,080	217,152	469	7.5
22	0	164	108	43	761,616	495,050	1069	10.3
23	+40	108	58	38	238,032	3,154,721	334	6.8
24	+180	92	63	44	255,024	165,766	358	5.8
25	+140	123	78	48	460,512	299,333	647	7.7
Average	140	84	48	33	170,951	111,118	240	5.3

Table A4. Quantification of boulder size, volume and estimated weight from CBB samples through Transect 4 at Ensenada Almeja. The laboratory result for density of banded rhyolite at 2.16 gm/cm³ is applied uniformly to all samples in this table.

Sample	Distance to Next (cm)	Long Axis (cm)	Intermediate Axis (cm)	Short Axis (cm)	Volume (cm³)	Adjust. to 65%	Weight (kg)	Estimated Wave ht. (m)
1	+700	50	30	19	28,500	18,525	40	3.1
2	0	48	18	16	13,824	89,896	19	3.0
3	+300	33	27	13	11,583	7529	16	2.1
4	+170	53	36	20	38,160	24,804	54	3.3
5	+160	40	25	12	12,000	7800	17	2.5
6	+190	44	27	14	16,632	10,810	23	2.8
7	+800	42	41	15	25,830	16,790	36	2.6
8	+600	38	38	30	43,320	28,158	61	2.4
9	+200	59	31	22	40,238	26,155	56	3.7
10	+110	52	30	25	39,000	23,350	50	3.3
11	0	62	44	19	51,832	33,691	73	3.9
12	+700	41	33	20	27,060	17,589	38	2.6
13	0	53	38	18	36,252	23,564	51	3.3
14	0	61	43	28	73,444	47,739	103	3.8
15	+900	63	32	29	58,464	38,002	82	4.0
16	0	67	48	42	135,072	87,797	190	4.2
17	+100	75	69	33	170,775	111,004	240	4.7
18	+20	71	30	23	48,990	31,844	69	4.5
19	0	58	33	18	34,452	22,394	48	3.6
20	+500	66	35	28	64,680	42,042	91	4.1
21	+200	60	42	20	50,400	32,760	71	3.8
22	0	59	35	16	33,040	21,476	46	3.7
23	0	68	33	28	62,832	40,841	88	4.3
24	+400	58	43	20	49,880	32,422	70	3.6
25	+20	63	39	28	68,796	44,717	97	4.0
Average	100	55	36	22	49,402	34,032	69	3.5

References

1. Muriá-Vila, D.; Jaimes, M.Á.; Pozos-Estrada, A.; López, A.; Reinoso, E.; Chávez, M.M.; Peña, F.; Sánchez-Sesma, J.; López, O. Effects of hurricane Odile on the infrastructure of Baja California Sur, Mexico. *Nat. Hazards* **2018**, *9*, 963–981. [CrossRef]
2. Johnson, M.E.; Ledesma-Vázquez, J.; Guardado-France, R. Coastal geomorphology of a Holocene hurricane deposit on a Pleistocene marine terrace from Isla Carmen (Baja California Sur, Mexico). *J. Mar. Sci. Eng.* **2018**, *6*, 108. [CrossRef]
3. Backus, D.H.; Johnson, M.E.; Ledesma-Vazquez, J. Peninsular and island rocky shores in the Gulf of California. In *Atlas of Coastal Ecosystems in the Western Gulf of California*; Johnson, M.E., Ledesma-Vazquez, J., Eds.; University Arizona Press: Tucson, Arizona, 2009; pp. 11–27. ISBN 978-0-8165-2530-0.

4. Stevens, E. A video clip showing storm activity below the Spanish Contessa's house at Ensendada San Basilio, CA, USA. Personal communication, 15 September 2014.
5. Ledesma-Vázquez, J.; Johnson, M.E.; Gonzalez-Yajimovich, O.; Santamaría-del-Angel, E. Gulf of California geography, geological origins, oceanography and sedimentation patterns. In *Atlas of Coastal Ecosystems in the Western Gulf of California*; Johnson, M.E., Ledesma-Vázquez, J., Eds.; University of Arizona Press: Tucson, AZ, USA, 2009; pp. 1–10. ISBN 978-0-8165-2530-0.
6. Backus, B.H.; Johnson, M.E. Sand dunes on peninsular and island shores in the Gulf of California. In *Atlas of Coastal Ecosystems in the Western Gulf of California*; Johnson, M.E., Ledesma-Vazquez, J., Eds.; University Arizona Press: Tucson, AZ, USA, 2009; pp. 117–133. ISBN 978-0-8165-2530-0.
7. Merrifield, M.A.; Winant, C.D. Shelf circulation in the Gulf of California: A description of the variability. *J. Geophy. Res.* **1989**, *94*, 133–160. [CrossRef]
8. Russell, P.; Johnson, M.E. Influence of seasonal winds on coastal carbonate dunes from the recent and Plio-Pleistocene at Punta Chivato (Baja California Sur, Mexico). *J. Coast. Res.* **2000**, *16*, 709–723.
9. Johnson, M.E.; Backus, D.H.; Carreño, A.L.; Ledesma-Vázquez, J. Rhyolite domes and subsequent offlap of Pliocene carbonates on volcanic islets at San Basilio (Baja California Sur, Mexico). *Geosciences* **2019**, *9*, 87. [CrossRef]
10. Wentworth, C.K. A scale of grade and class terms for clastic sediments. *J. Geol.* **1922**, *27*, 377–392. [CrossRef]
11. Ruban, D.A.; Ponedelnik, A.A.; Yashalova, N.N. Megaclasts: Term use and relevant biases. *Geosciences* **2019**, *9*, 14. [CrossRef]
12. Sneed, E.D.; Folk, R.L. Pebbles in the lower Colorado River of Texas: A study in particle morphogenesis. *J. Geol.* **1958**, *66*, 114–150. [CrossRef]
13. Nott, J. Waves, coastal bolder deposits and the importance of pre-transport setting. *Earth Planet. Sci. Lett.* **2003**, *210*, 269–276. [CrossRef]
14. Paz-Moreno, F.; Demant, A. The recent Isla San Luis volcanic center: Petrology of a rift-related volcanic suite in the northern Gulf of California, Mexico. *J. Volcanol. Geotherm. Res.* **1999**, *93*, 31–52. [CrossRef]
15. Scutter, C.R.; Cas, R.A.F.; Moore, C.L. Facies architecture and origin of a submarine rhyolitic lava flow-dome complex, Ponza, Italy. *J. Geophys. Res. Solid Earth* **1998**, *103*, 551–566. [CrossRef]
16. Calanchi, N.; De Rosa, R.; Mazzuoli, R.; Rossi, R.; Santacroce, R.; Ventura, G. Silicic magma entering a basaltic magma chamber: Eruptive dynamics and magma mizing—an example from Salina (Aeolian islands, Southern Tyrrhenian Sea). *Bull. Volcanol.* **1993**, *55*, 504–522. [CrossRef]
17. Hayes, M.L.; Johnson, M.E.; Fox, W.T. Rocky-shore biotic associations and their fossilization potential: Isla Requeson (Baja California Sur, Mexico). *J. Coast. Res.* **1993**, *9*, 944–957.
18. Avila-Serrano, G.E.; Téllez-Duarte, M.A.; Flessa, K.W. Ecological changes on the Colorado River Delta: The Shelley Fauna Evidence. In *Atlas of Coastal Ecosystems in the Western Gulf of California*; Johnson, M.E., Ledesma-Vazquez, J., Eds.; University Arizona Press: Tucson, AZ, USA, 2009; pp. 95–103. ISBN 978-0-8165-2530-0.
19. Ramírez-Herrera, M.-T.; Lagos, M.; Hutchinson, I.; Kostoglodov, V.; Machain, M.L.; Caballero, M.; Coguitchaichvili, A.; Aguilar, B.; Cagué-Goff, C.; Goff, J.; et al. Extreme wave deposits on the Pacific coast of Mexico: Tsunamis or storms? A multi-proxy approach. *Geomorphology* **2012**, *139*, 360–371. [CrossRef]
20. Trejo-Gómez, E.; Ortiz, M.; Núñez-Cornú, J. Source model of the October 9, 1995 Jalisco-Colima tsunami as constrained by field survey reports and on the numerical simulation of the tsunami. *Geofís. Int.* **2015**, *54*, 149–159. [CrossRef]
21. Ramalho, R.S.; Winckler, G.; Madeira, J.; Helffrich, G.R.; Hipólito, A.; Quartau, R.; Adena, K.; Schaefer, J.M. Hazard potential of volcanic flank collapses raised by new megatsuanmi evidence. *Sci. Adv.* **2015**, *1*, e1500456. [CrossRef]
22. Romero-Vadillo, E.; Zaystev, O.; Morales-Pérez, R. Tropical cyclone statistics in the northeastern Pacific. *Atmósfera* **2007**, *20*, 197–213.
23. Backus, D.H.; Johnson, M.E.; Riosmena-Rodríguez, R. Distribution, sediment source and costal erosion of fan-delta systems on Isla Cerralvo (lower Gulf of California, Mexico). *J. Coast. Res.* **2012**, *28*, 210–224. [CrossRef]
24. Kozlowski, J.A.; Johnson, M.E.; Ledesma-Vázquez, J.; Birgel, D.; Peckmann, J.; Schleper, C. Microbial diversity of a closed salt lagoon in the Puertecitos area, Upper Gulf of California. *Cienc. Mar.* **2018**, *44*, 71–90. [CrossRef]

25. Ledesma-Vázquez, J.; Johnson, M.E.; Backus, D.H.; Mirabal-Davila, C. Coastal evolution from transgressive barrier deposit to marine terrace on Isla Coronados, Baja California Sur, Mexico. *Cienc. Mar.* **2007**, *33*, 335–351. [CrossRef]
26. Johnson, M.E.; Ledesma-Vázquez, J. Biological zonation on a rocky-shore boulder deposit: Upper Pleistocene Bahía San Antonio (Baja California Sur, Mexico). *Palaios* **1999**, *14*, 569–584. [CrossRef]
27. Johnson, M.E.; Ledesma-Vázquez, J.; Backus, D.H.; González, M.R. Lagoon microbialites on Isla Angel de la Guarda and associated peninsular shores, Gulf of California (Mexico). *Sediment. Geol.* **2012**, *263*, 76–84. [CrossRef]
28. Cox, R.; Jahn, K.L.; Watkins, O.G.; Cox, P. Extraordinary boulder transport by storm waves (west Ireland, winter 2013-14) and criteria for analyzing coastal boulder deposits. *Earth-Sci. Rev.* **2018**, *177*, 623–636. [CrossRef]
29. Hearty, P.J. Boulder deposits from large waves during the last inter-glaciation on North Eleuthera Island, Bahamas. *Quat. Res.* **1997**, *48*, 326–338. [CrossRef]
30. Rovere, A.; Casella, E.; Harris, D.L.; Lorscheid, T.; Nandasena, N.A.K.; Dyer, B.; Sandstrom, M.R.; Stocchi, P.; D'Amdrea, W.J.; Raymo, M.E. Giant boulders and last interglacial storm intensity in the North Atlantic. *Proc. Natl. Acad. Sci. USA* **2017**, *114*, 12144–12149. [CrossRef] [PubMed]
31. Biolchi, S.; Furlani, S.; Devoto, S.; Scicchitano, G.; Korbar, T.; Vilibic, I.; Sepic, J. The origin and dynamics of coastal boulders in a semi-enclosed shallow basin: A northern Adriatic case study. *Mar. Geol.* **2019**, *411*, 62–77. [CrossRef]

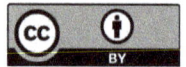

© 2019 by the authors. Licensee MDPI, Basel, Switzerland. This article is an open access article distributed under the terms and conditions of the Creative Commons Attribution (CC BY) license (http://creativecommons.org/licenses/by/4.0/).

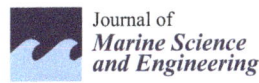

Article

Mathematical Modeling Framework of Physical Effects Induced by Sediments Handling Operations in Marine and Coastal Areas

Iolanda Lisi [1,*,†], Alessandra Feola [1,†], Antonello Bruschi [1,†], Andrea Pedroncini [2,†], Davide Pasquali [3,†] and Marcello Di Risio [1,3,†]

1. Italian National Institute for Environmental Protection and Research (ISPRA), 00144 Rome, Italy; alessandra.feola@isprambiente.it (A.F.); antonello.bruschi@isprambiente.it (A.B.); marcello.dirisio@univaq.it (M.D.R.)
2. DHI S.r.l., 16149 Genova, Italy; anp@dhigroup.com
3. Department of Civil, Construction-Architectural and Environmental Engineering (DICEAA)—Environmental and Maritime Hydraulic Laboratory (LIam), University of L'Aquila, 67100 L'Aquila, Italy; davide.pasquali@univaq.it
* Correspondence: iolanda.lisi@isprambiente.it; Tel.: +39-650074653
† These authors contributed equally to this work.

Received: 27 March 2019; Accepted: 10 May 2019; Published: 15 May 2019

Abstract: In recent years increasing attention has been paid to environmental effects that may result from marine dredging and disposal operations. In general, the fine-grained fraction of handled sediments can be dispersed far from the intervention site as a turbidity plume, depending on the specific site and operational parameters. Starting from a literature review, this paper suggests standards for estimating and characterizing the sediment source term, for setting up far-field modeling studies and analyzing numerical results, with the aim of optimizing, also from an economic point of view, the different project, execution and monitoring phases. The paper proposes an integrated modeling approach for simulating sediment dispersion due to sediment handling operations in different marine-coastal areas (off-shore, near-shore and semi-enclosed basins). Attention is paid to the characterization of sediment source terms due to different operational phases (removal, transport and disposal). The paper also deals with the definition of accuracy level of modeling activities, with regard to the main physical processes characterizing the different marine–coastal areas and to the type of environmental critical issues near the intervention site (if any). The main relationships between modeling and monitoring are given for the different design and management phases to support the selection of appropriate technical alternatives and monitoring actions and to ensure the environmental compliance of the proposed interventions.

Keywords: dredging and disposal; environmental effects; mathematical modeling and monitoring; sediment dispersion; sediment handling

1. Introduction

Interventions in marine and coastal areas often involve sediment dredging and disposal operations. The volume of sediments handling can vary in relation to the operations purposes, e.g., to maintain or improve the navigation depth of ports and harbors (e.g., [1]), for creating or improving facilities (e.g., [2]), for beach nourishment (e.g., [3]) and open-water disposal (e.g., [4]), to carefully remove and relocate contaminated materials (e.g., [5]) or morphological reconstruction in transitional areas. Moreover, the operational techniques (e.g., type and capacity of dredges) are key aspects to be accounted for when dealing with the assessment of physical effects due to sediment handling works (e.g., [6,7]).

Pre-approval from controlling authorities is typically required to verify environmental and economic compatibility of equipment, work plans and operational criteria prior to the initiation of the activities. The approval requirements include the evaluation of short-term effects occurring during the project phases (often referred to as process effects) and long-term effects caused by the final project layout (often referred to as project effects, e.g., [8]).

For the European Union, detailed environmental impact assessment (Directive 2014/52/UE, [9]) are aimed at selecting technical alternatives and designing appropriate mitigation measures and monitoring actions for ensuring environmental compliance, especially when either large quantities or polluted sediments have to be handled. Far from the intervention areas the dispersal and settling of plumes of spilled sediment can induce a broad range of effects, i.e., light reduction and sedimentation at sensitive receptors, changes in abundance, diversity and biomass of seabed habitats and benthic communities, contaminants and nutrients release. An efficient management of sediment handling works requires knowledge both of the operational factors (i.e., extension of dredging/disposal areas, kinematic and geometric parameters of dredging/disposal techniques, duration and timing of operations) to assess the sediment release mechanisms, and of the site conditions (i.e., sediment type, water depth, currents and waves climates, thermohaline stratification, seasonal window) to assess the spatial dispersion and the settling time of the sediment plume during and after the end of operations.

In this framework, mathematical models are recognized as a valuable tool to forecast the plume dynamics and the areas interested by significant variations of suspended sediment concentration (SSC) and sediment deposition rates (DEP, e.g., [10–12]). Recent research (e.g., [13]) and international guidelines (e.g., [14]) often include the use of mathematical models to perform environmental studies needed to support decision makers (before, during and after execution) to optimize the interventions and monitoring actions with regard to environmental and project objectives [15], while maintaining desired production rates [16]. A major effort has been put to support contractors and controlling authorities to combine modeling and monitoring activities in a feedback framework [15,17,18]. This is aimed (i) at assessing and approving dredging equipment and work plans (prior to the operations start), and (ii) at introducing assessment procedures based on the application of environmental criteria, for ensuring that SSC remains below specified limits (during the operations) and for timely changing work plans and monitoring frequencies to prevent any potential short- and long-term environmental effects (during and after the operations).

Common modeling approaches involves hydrodynamic and transport models suitable to quantify and to compare the transport processes of the different spilled sediment, moving from the near- to the far-field (e.g., [11,12,19,20]). Nevertheless, technical and scientific literature highlights the lack of an organic and comprehensive methodology driving the selection of appropriate modeling tools and of accuracy levels needed for a reliable assessment of the induced physical effects in different environmental contexts and when environmental critical issues are involved (e.g., ecological sensitive receptor, water quality, sensitive habitat and species, fish farming facilities, regulatory constraints, etc.). In the context of national experiences, the Italian National Institute for Environmental Protection and Research (ISPRA) issued the Italian Guidelines dealing with the modeling approach that can be implemented in relation both to environmental and project objectives, promoting uniform procedures for different techniques, operational phases, and environmental contexts [15].

For ensuring the compliance with environmental requirements, the selection of a modeling approach must balance the accuracy of results related to strict environmental critical issues and operating criteria defined prior the initiations of the operations. Moreover, input data for the selected modeling scenarios should be appropriate for a reliable representation of the main physical processes variability driving the dynamic of the plume during the different operational phases, depending on the main characteristics of the selected techniques. It has to be stressed that past studies (e.g., [14,21,22]) found that results rarely focus on long-term effects of sediments dispersion, within either seasonal or annual time windows. Rather, they are focused on short-term scenarios usually related to either one or few tidal cycles or extreme events (e.g., [23–25]).

Increases of SSC and DEP away from the re-suspension source are mainly used to evaluate the extension of the area affected by plume dispersion, where the maximum SSC is usually expressed in relation to given thresholds. It has to be stressed that there is also a lack of tools that synthesize and make the modeling results useful for supporting decision system and environmental management [22] and to give operational and environmental indications to optimize all the planning and management phases of the sediment handling project.

GBRMPA [14] and Feola et al. [26] recommend that model results should be synthesized by means of maps showing statistical measures (i.e., maximum and mean) of the predicted SSC and DEP at different water depths, as well as by the synthetic parameters of the time series at different key sites, intended to be representative of the environmental context and of the duration of the project. It is suggested to analyze environmental effects in terms of the duration of the time windows during which given SSC thresholds are exceeded during the operations [16].

Starting from a literature review, this paper suggests standards for both setting up modeling and field studies and for analyzing and assessing modeling results with regards to: (i) areas of intervention (coastal areas, semi-enclosed basins and offshore areas), (ii) operational phases (excavation, loading/transport and disposal), (iii) operational techniques (hydraulic and mechanical dredges), and (iv) environmentally sensitive critical issues (if any). For sake of clarity, the key points of this paper are:

- an organic and comprehensive framework about the physical effects induced by sediments handling operations is proposed;
- a broad-spectrum modeling approach intended to support contractors and controlling authorities in planning and managing sediment handling operations is detailed;
- an integrated, flexible and replicable methodological approach for synthesizing numerical results is illustrated;
- the main features of the required modeling–monitoring feedback system are highlighted.

This paper is structured as follows. Section 2 aims at describing the proposed methodological approach. Sections 3 and 4 detail the rationale for the selection of scenarios and the source term definition respectively. Sections 5 and 6 illustrate the proposed integrated modeling approach for simulating sediment dispersion, intended as a general framework to assess the physical effects of sediments handling operation, thus by identifying areas interested by significant changes in terms of physical parameters (e.g., SSC and DEP) due to plume dynamics, and from which environmental risk can be derived. Also, the relationship between modeling and monitoring activities for proper implementation and verification both of modeling studies and of decision processes in different project phases are outlined (Section 8.1), and the importance of the management and sharing of monitoring data is highlighted (Section 8.2). Concluding remarks close the paper.

2. The Proposed Modeling Approach

This paper provides an organic and comprehensive framework about the physical effects induced by sediments handling operations and proposes a broad-spectrum modeling approach intended to support contractors and controlling authorities in planning and managing such a kind of interventions. Hereinafter, the plume dynamics are intended to be related either to removal or disposal induced re-suspension/release of the fine fraction of the handled sediments, as well as to advection, deposition and sometimes re-suspension from the bottom due to environmental forcing. The whole sediment handling work cycle is described by different operational phases: removal (or excavation), loading, transport and disposal of handled sediments. Moreover, different environmental contexts (coastal areas, semi-enclosed basins and offshore areas) are considered as intervention areas.

Even if the water depth, respectively in shallow or deep offshore areas, may induce operational differences in excavation and disposal, these distinctions are not addressed in this paper. Indeed, as also suggested by Marine Strategy Framework Directive 2008/56/EC [27], the area of interest should be defined taking into account the strict interaction between off-shore and near-shore hydrodynamics. Then, the area of interest could reach the national limits and beyond, of course with an appropriate and feasible spatial scale. Hence, all the main physical phenomena influencing the dynamics of the induced sediment plumes can be properly modeled.

Mathematical models, calibrated and validated through the use of literature and field data, are recognized as useful supporting tools to plan, design and manage sediment handling operations. In particular, they can support the comparative choice of the technical and operational alternatives based on the forecast of possible environmental issues. The reliable estimation of the physical processes characterizing the sediment plume dynamic during the whole handling cycle requires the selection of mathematical models able to reproduce the primary physical features of the intervention area, of the project goals, and of the environmental aspects. The proper model selection and implementation require the definition of the main hydrodynamic field and source term features driving the spatial and temporal variability of dispersal of the spilled sediment and contamination processes (if any). Similarly, the selected approach for the numerical solution of the governing equations for hydrodynamic and transport phenomena influences the burden in terms of resources, computational times and of required input data.

The proposed integrated modeling approach relies on standard numerical suites worldwide used to model the passive phase of plume dispersion, but the source term definition aimed at accounting for the near-field processes, at least from a macro-scale point of view. Three numerical modules, hereinafter referred to as the hydrodynamic module (H-M in Figure 1), source term module (ST-M in Figure 1) and transport module (T-M in Figure 1) are implemented in series. Basically, the transport module is used to estimate SSC and DEP resulting from dispersion of the sediment release (estimated by the source term module) due to the flow field variability (estimated by the hydrodynamic module). Then, an environmental assessment module (EA-M in Figure 1) provides standard methods and statistical parameters for the assessment of the physical environmental effects. A modeling–monitoring feedback system is then recommended and considered as an integral part of the proposed integrated modeling approach. With the aim to define a proper modeling setup, validation of modeling results and verifying when sediment spill exceeds specified limits. These limits, hereinafter referred to as reference levels, are intended to be defined with respect to the natural background conditions and to the environmental critical issues types (if any).

Lisi et al. [15] suggest that the modeling studies should be performed in different steps, with increasing level of detail, and they give practical indications to optimize the work plan, with regard to environmental and operational site-specific objectives. The accuracy of quantitative estimates depends on the used modeling approach (modeling tools and scenarios), and it is a function of the expected results. Indeed, depending on the project phase (i.e., prior, during or after), different detail levels can be required. Furthermore, this also makes the proposed methodology feasible from an economic point of view (Figure 2). It is argued that expert judgment should be the first effort performed. A preliminary information phase aims at selecting reference conditions to assess when modeling approaches are needed and to define their accuracy level with respect to environmental expected effects. Within this phase, based on operative and environmental data collection, scientists with different expertise should be engaged within the framework of a holistic approach. When the preliminary information phase highlights that significant environmental effects are likely to occur, the implementation of modeling studies is recommended for their estimation. In these cases, the next step is the implementation of a preliminary modeling phase, in which simplified models are used to describe the key features of the plume dynamic and allow a fast estimation of its expected maximum extension area. The reader is referred to Section 5 for details on preliminary information phase and preliminary modeling phase. A detailed modeling phase (see Section 6 for details) is then suggested when the preliminary modeling phase confirms that the dispersion of spilled sediment can impact on water quality and on the site-specific environmental targets. It is intended to allow accurate evaluations even for complex conditions.

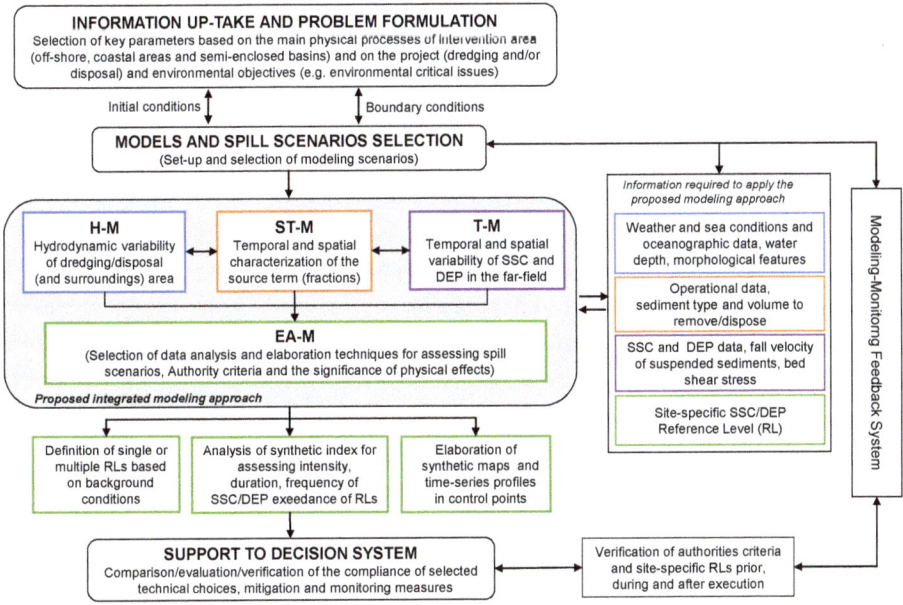

Figure 1. Flow chart of the proposed methodological approach.

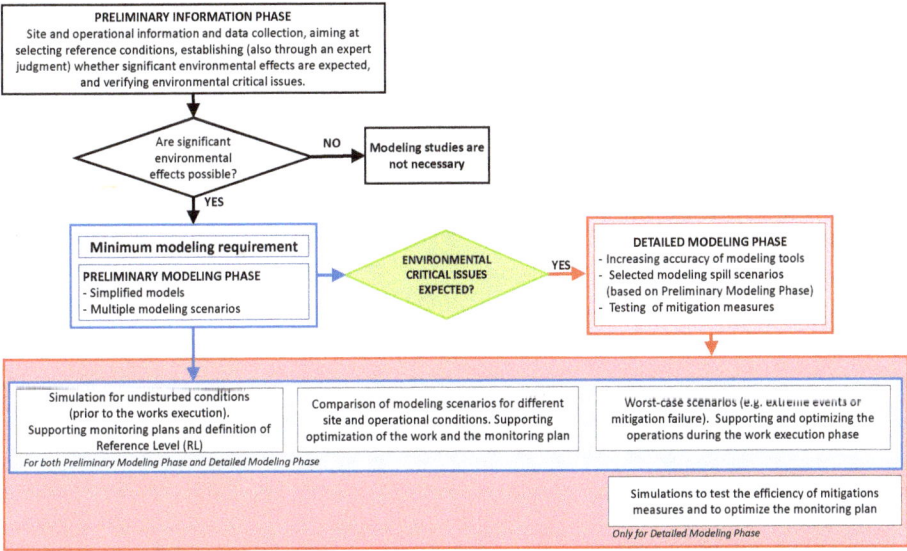

Figure 2. Flow chart of the different phases suggested for optimizing the modeling studies (thus the work plan and the related monitoring) to be performed with increasing level of detail during the different project phases.

The detailed modeling phase is always recommended when three-dimensional features (for source terms and/or hydrodynamic patterns) play a key role and when environmental critical issues are revealed and/or predicted by preliminary modeling phase. It has to be stressed that the preliminary modeling phase plays an important role even when detailed modeling is implemented, in order to evaluate the possible need and the nature of detailed analysis and to support the preliminary assessment of the worst-case scenarios (e.g., extreme events or mitigation failure). This is aimed at optimizing the work plan and the approval procedures, with regard to environmental and operational site-specific objectives. Figure 2 depicts the flow chart of the proposed general approach.

Some initial modeling assumptions (e.g., within the preliminary information phase and preliminary modeling phase) may vary during the project development (e.g., from the planning phase up to the execution). Indeed, it may be observed that key information could not well defined at the preliminary design phase of a sediment handling project, while it is (or should be at least) known at a later stage. According to the adaptive management approach [17], a stepwise procedure can address uncertainties as the project progresses, incorporating flexibility and robustness into project design, and using latest information to instruct decision-makers as the project develops.

3. Scenarios

The selection of the scenarios to be modeled plays a crucial role in the choice of the mathematical models and also on the reliability of the modeling results obtained for the relevant physical phenomena.

Herein, four different modeling scenarios are proposed and detailed for driving the proper implementation of the proposed integrated modeling approach (Table 1): climatological, short-term realistic, long-term realistic and operational/forecasting scenarios.

The climatological approach allows reproducing conditions which are not directly related to a specific series of measured data. They are inferred from observations by means of statistical analysis on available data. The aim is to reproduce either frequent (annual or seasonal) or extreme conditions with given average return periods. It should be stressed that statistical analysis seldom allows defining the return levels of relevant driving forces by taking into account also the marginal probability, i.e., that extreme events of different forcing may occur simultaneously. Usually, this approach is used within the frame of the preliminary modeling phase, when most of the information or data are not available yet.

The shortcoming of the climatological approach may be overcome by employing the short-term realistic approach that considers actually observed driving forces for a short duration time window (event scale). Then, it is possible to take into account the interaction of all driving processes typical of real conditions that can significantly affect the actual dynamics. This method is suitable within the frame of both preliminary information phase and preliminary modeling phase, and detailed modeling phase as well. In the preliminary phases, it allows achieving results with low computational costs useful to depict the big picture of the problem at hand when critical conditions are analyzed. In the detailed phases, it can be considered for either validation purposes or to reproduce extreme events observed in the past. It has to be stressed that this approach may be employed only when detailed measurements are available.

The long-term realistic approach has to be used when long-term effects (or project effects) have to be investigated within the framework of the detailed modeling phase. The definition of the long-term scenarios is then based on real conditions which occurred in the past, for a long duration time window selected as representative of the site-specific conditions. Hence, long-term time series (i.e., years) have to be available by means of either monitoring activities or numerical hindcast (e.g., [28]). The long-term realistic approach allows investigating the probability of exceeding thresholds for the variables of interest (e.g., SSC, see Section 8.1) in terms of combined analysis of intensity, duration and frequency.

During the works execution the operational/forecasting approach can be employed to forecast worst scenarios (in term of weather and sea conditions, and sediment dispersion conditions), within the framework of the environmental monitoring plan. This method can be useful for contractors to optimize the work execution. Indeed, safe conditions may be forecast hours or days in advance (e.g., [29]). Moreover, authorities need to make effective the implementation of the environmental monitoring plan and then to limit environmental effects within the framework of the modeling–monitoring feedback system (see Section 8.1).

Table 1 synthesizes the main features of the four approaches for scenarios selection needed to implement the proposed integrated modeling approach.

Table 1. Main features of the modeling scenarios proposed within the different accuracy levels of the proposed integrated approach.

Approach	Aim	Limitations	Needed Data
Climatological	To reproduce specific conditions not directly related to measured data, e.g., to specific Average Return Period.	The marginal occurrence probability (i.e., simultaneity of driving forces) is seldom reproduced.	Results of statistical analyses (e.g., of either atmospheric or hydrodynamic forcing).
Short-term realistic	To reproduce specific conditions observed in the past in order to take into account the simultaneity of different driving forces. The results can be used for numerical models validation.	The needed data are seldom available, in particular during the preliminary modeling phase.	Observed or hindcast short-duration time series.
Long-term realistic	To reproduce the long-term response of the system related to the project effects evaluation. A statistical analysis of the results is possible.	The long-term time series have to be representative of the variability of the driving forces, i.e., they should be related to both frequent and extreme conditions.	Observed or hindcast long-duration time series.
Operational/ forecasting	To reproduce the short-term evolution of the system during the works within the frame of a real-time optimization of the works.	A specific infrastructure should be foreseen in order to promptly provide the Contractors with updated forecast of the system evolution.	Forecast data.

4. Source Term Definition

Efficient management of sediment handling operations requires sufficient knowledge of dredging and disposal methods and of main mechanisms of release that can affect the SSC transport processes for different excavation and disposal techniques. The selection of spill scenarios is a key factor for environmental assessment and approval of the work plans. Indeed, it influences the source term needed as input to far field models.

In particular, the temporal and spatial characterization of the source term is important for the comparison, on different spatial and temporal scales, of scenarios with the least probabilities of detrimental impacts on water quality and to define whether (and when) mitigation measures should be taken on future work plans (e.g., [30]). This paper is aimed at estimating the contribution to source terms of phenomena directly related to marine sediment handling activities. However, sedimentation processes and the related re-suspension of the sediment due to hydrodynamic agitation (waves and currents) can have a significant influence on the magnitude of the source terms and therefore on the sediment transport modeling (see Section 6). Some mathematical models do not explicitly include the modeling of sedimentation and re-suspension related to hydrodynamic agitation. Nevertheless, their knowledge (or monitoring) may be crucial when the choice of the type and mode of implementation of the models is concerned. Moreover, also the definition of the background (baseline) conditions for the parameters of interest (e.g., SSC and turbidity), needed to identify the related single or multiple site-specifics reference levels, can be related to the sedimentation and re-suspension related to hydrodynamic agitation.

Basically, two main approaches may be used to model the flux of fine sediments available to the far field dispersion. Computational fluid dynamics (CFD) framework may be used for detailing near-field regimes and then to get a reliable estimate of the mechanisms that govern the dynamic of the sediment fraction leaving the re-suspension/release area as a passive (dispersive) plume. Such an approach has large computational costs and the results may be hardly generalized. On the other hand, a second approach may be used within the frame of macro-scale modeling (i.e., conceptual or empirical models). A series of empirical and numerical near-field models to estimate the suspended sediment flux leaving the intervention area have been developed so far (e.g., [6,8,31–35]).

A few conceptual models to predict the resuspended sediment mass rate at the resuspension point, and thus its source strength and geometry, have been proposed for dredging actitivies (e.g., [6,31,33,34], see Lisi et al. [13] for a comprehensive review). They give an estimate of source term as a function of the site (i.e., sediment properties, water depth, currents) and operational (i.e., dredge type, dredge-head dimension) parameters.

As suggested by John et al. [30] and recalled by Becker et al. [8], the source term may be estimated either (i) by looking at the sediment concentration increase at the re-suspension area (e.g., [6]), or (ii) by providing the sediment release rate at the re-suspension area (e.g., [6]), or (iii) by taking advantage of the definition of the S-factor (e.g., [31,34]) that gives the estimate of the released sediments as a fraction of the total mass of handled sediments, or (iv) by providing the sediment flux across the area bounding the re-suspension zone (e.g., [6]). All these approaches are hard to be used in a generalized way as they are site- and operation-dependent. Indeed, the available conceptual methods for estimating the source term induced by different re-suspension sources are based on the use of tabular data, e.g., the turbidity generation unit (TGU) approach proposed by Nakai [31] and the re-suspension factor proposed by Hayes et al. [34]. On the other hand, the use of empirical formulations involve sets of dimensionless parameters related to operating and site characteristics (e.g., [6,33,36]).

As for dredging activities, a few conceptual models exist also for other sediment handling works (e.g., either open water disposal [4,35] or beach nourishments [37]).

In order to overcome the lack of engineering tools, Becker et al. [8] proposed a general approach able to provide the estimation of source term. Basically, they suggest to estimate the amount of fine-graded sediments and to distribute the release into the water column after an in-depth analysis of possible plume sources. Hence, for each phase (excavation, loading/transport and disposal) of the considered handling work, it is possible to estimate a specific source term fraction to be used as input for the far-field model if it is properly applied on the computational grid. It can be observed that this approach perfectly suits the approach proposed herein.

The results of specific in-situ analyses on the sediments to be handled allows estimating the quantity of fine-graded fraction available to the far field. The fraction expressed by either R_{74} (the fraction of sediments with grain diameter lower than 74 µm as per the fine-sediments definition of the unified soil classification system, e.g., [6]) or R_{63} (the fraction of sediments with grain diameter lower than 63 µm as per the Wentworth scale, e.g., [8]) may be used to estimate the fine sediments mass (m_f) available to the far field (e.g., [8]):

$$m_f = \rho_d V_t R_f \qquad (1)$$

where ρ_d is the dry density of the in situ material, V_t is the handled volume of sediments and R_f is the considered fine fraction (either R_{74} or R_{63}). The dry mass of fine sediment released into the water column (m_r) can be then easily estimated by using a series of empirical parameters (σ):

$$m_r = \sigma m_f. \qquad (2)$$

Becker et al. [8] (see their Table 1) provide reasonable values of the empirical source term fraction (i.e., σ) for drag-head induced re-suspension ($\sigma = 0.00$–0.03), overflow induced re-suspension ($\sigma = 0.00$–0.20), cutter-head induced re-suspension ($\sigma = 0.00$–0.04), spill from mechanical dredging ($\sigma = 0.00$–0.04), disposal by bottom door either mechanical ($\sigma = 0.00$–0.10) or hydraulic ($\sigma = 0.00$–0.05). It has to be stressed that the definition of the empirical source term fractions may take advantage of either monitoring activities or empirical formulations. Just as an example, Hayes et al. [33] proposed an empirical formulation aimed at estimating the rate of sediment (r) re-suspended by cutterhead dredge as a fraction of sediment mass dredged:

$$r = \frac{(L_c d_c)^{1.966} |V_s \pm \pi d_c \alpha|^{1.966} (V_s A_E)^{1.804}}{1.099 Q^{3.770}}, \quad (3)$$

where r (%) is the fraction of sediment mass dredged expressed as a percentage (hence intimately related to the source term fraction $\sigma_c = r/100$), L_c (m) is the length of the cutterhead, d_c (m) is the cutter diameter, V_s (m/s) is the swing velocity, α (rounds per second) is the rotational speed of the cutter, A_E (m^2) is the total surface area exposed to washing, Q (m^3/s) is the volumetric flow rate into the dredge pipe. If overcutting is considered (i.e., the positive sign is used in the numerator of Equation (3)), Figure 3 shows the estimate of the empirical source term fraction σ_c for varying swing velocity (V_s) and varying rotation speed of the cutter (α) for a typical 16-in. (0.41 m) dredge (e.g., [33], $d_c = 1.07$ m, $L_c = 0.91$ m, $A_E \simeq 1.3$ m^2). It could be observed that the empirical source term fraction proposed by Becker et al. [8] (dashed areas in Figure 3) is of the same order of magnitude given by the more detailed empirical formulation by Hayes et al. [33].

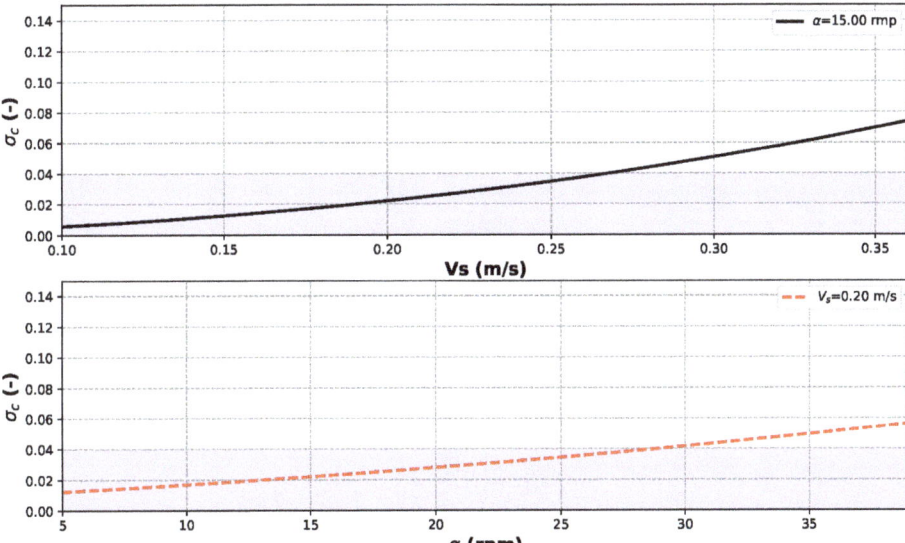

Figure 3. Empirical source term fraction (σ_c) for cutter-head induced re-suspension as a function of the swing speed (V_s, upper panel) and of the rotational speed of the cutter (α, lower panel) as estimated on the basis of the model proposed by Hayes et al. [33]. Shaded areas highlight the range suggested by Becker et al. [8].

It has to be noticed that Equation (2) gives the mass of fine sediments available to the far field. In order to get the correct estimate of the source term, a sediment flux should be provided. Then, Becker et al. [8] suggest to simply divide the mass m_r by the time duration of the considered phase (i.e., either excavation, transport, or disposal). This highlights the importance of the analysis of the work phases. This is equally crucial when dealing with the timing and the location of the source term within the computational domain (see Section 5, Figures 4 and 5). Indeed, depending on the operational parameters of the handling works, the source term can be described by either a time-varying or constant intensity and by either a time-varying or fixed location. On the other hand, depending on the spatial resolution of the study, the source term can be described by either a punctual or a finite extent re-suspension source.

Figure 4 aims at synthesizing the main features of the source term estimation and how it can be applied to the computational domain.

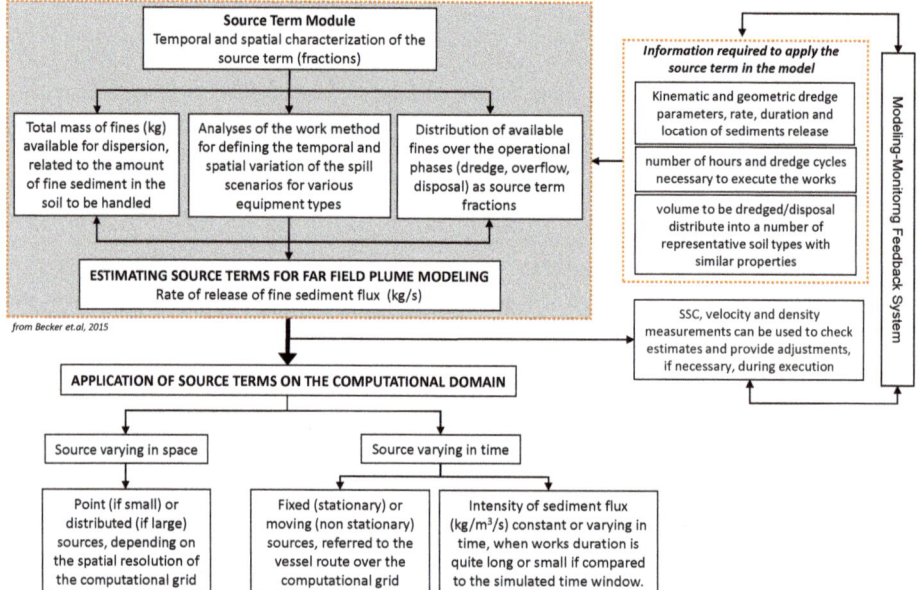

Figure 4. Main steps of the source term module for both the estimation and the application of the source term in the computational domain.

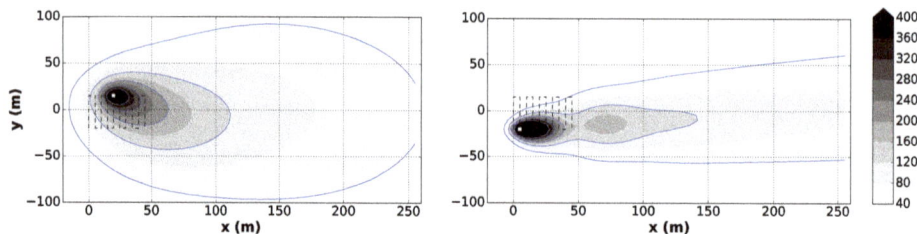

Figure 5. Analytical solution obtained by using the model proposed by Di Risio et al. [39]. Typical examples for hydraulic dredging (**left**) and mechanical dredging (**right**) are shown. Constant velocity along x-direction is considered. Dashed lines depict the dredge-head path during the works execution, square markers indicate the instantaneous location of the dredge-head. Color scale refers to the suspended sediment concentration (SSC) (g/m^3).

5. Preliminary Information and Modeling Phases

The modeling approach has to be feasible both from the controlling authorities point of view, that need reliable results to avoid, or at least to minimize, detrimental effects on the environment, and from the contractors point of view that have to pay attention to the economic and technical feasibility of the work.

Within the framework of the preliminary information phase, the preliminary analysis should be devoted to identifying the need of more detailed studies to prevent and/or mitigate the expected environmental effects.

The first and more basic preliminary studies are based on the retrieval and analyses of known data about environmental forcing (i.e., mainly related to hydrodynamics) along with the physical features of handled sediments (i.e., fine fraction). This approach allows gaining insight into the big picture of the phenomena at hand by identifying potential environmental effects. Environmental issues have to be identified within the frame of a holistic approach, hence by engaging scientists with different expertise (e.g., [38]). Of course, this phase has strong limitations and needs a more detailed analysis if significant environmental effects are expected to occur. In this way, the probability of detrimental environmental effects identified within the preliminary information phase may be confirmed. If this is the case, a second (and deeper) level of modeling to get reliable expectation in terms of turbidity plume evolution and deposition rate distribution at and around the work site should be then performed.

When preliminary modeling phase is concerned, the synthetic scenarios approach is considered the proper candidate to provide fast results. Despite their limitations, analytical models can be used to provide modeling results taking into account the main features of the phenomenon with low computational costs. The solutions of the (simplified) governing equations are typically given in closed-form (they require simple arithmetic operations) or integral-form (they require standard numerical integration techniques). Simplified models for sediment transport and deposition rate estimates often rely on the solution of the two-dimensional advection and diffusion equation of the re-suspended sediments that reads as follow (e.g., [39]):

$$\frac{\partial C}{\partial t} + U\frac{\partial C}{\partial x} + V\frac{\partial C}{\partial y} + \frac{\partial}{\partial x}\left(D_x\frac{\partial C}{\partial x}\right) + \frac{\partial}{\partial y}\left(D_y\frac{\partial C}{\partial y}\right) = q - \frac{w_s}{h}C, \tag{4}$$

where x and y are the horizontal coordinates; t is the elapsed time; C is the depth-averaged sediments concentration (intimately related to the SSC); U and V are the x- and y-component of the ambient current respectively; D_x and D_y are the diffusion coefficients; w_s is the settling velocity; h is the water depth; q is the source term, often referred to as re-suspension source strength (e.g., [6]). The latter is intended to describe the sediments actually available to the far-field passive transport (see Section 4). Equation (4) neglects the vertical variability of SSC. These models also consider homogeneous environmental currents (i.e., not variable in space), even if variable over time, homogeneous and constant diffusion coefficients (albeit with the possibility of simulating anisotropy of the medium and of the flow), constant depth and constant settling velocity. It is therefore clear that these models can only be used within the preliminary modeling phase, in which simplified models can in any case describe salient features of the spatial and temporal evolution of the plume, and thus highlight when environmental critical issues can potentially occur.

As far as the source term is concerned, analytical models are usually able to evaluate the evolution of the turbidity plume with a constant production of sediments over time located in a fixed area (often referred to as continuous source, e.g., [40,41]). Nevertheless, analytical models can take into account the variation, in both time and space, of location and strength of the re-suspension source during the work progression (e.g., [39]). Thus, it is possible to provide the temporal and spatial picture of the resulting plume evolution. Figure 5 shows a typical example obtained by using the analytical approach proposed by Di Risio et al. ([39]) in the case of dredging activities performed with a hydraulic dredge and a mechanical dredge. In the former case (left panel), the re-suspension is modeled as a moving and continuous source with varying intensity. In the latter (right panel), the re-suspension is modeled as a moving and intermittent source.

Even with their strong limitations, analytical models were demonstrated to be able for describing the big picture of the phenomenon at hand [39] and for the comparison of the effects for different scenarios. Therefore, they can be used to address the general environmental questions, allowing a first rough estimation of the maximum impacted area. Indeed, this is useful to guide more detailed numerical analysis and to select the more appropriate simulation scenarios in terms of both environmental forcing and operational techniques.

6. Detailed Modeling Phase

6.1. Hydrodynamic Modeling

Within the detailed modeling phase, hydrodynamics plays a crucial role. The selection of the models type and the accuracy levels of the modeling scenarios should be representative of the project-specific features and of the spatial and temporal scales of the main physical processes driving the sediment transport phenomena. Then, the analysis has to be based on the environmental conditions of the intervention site: the complexity of the models implies the knowledge about forcing terms and the geometry of the site.

Basically, the hydrodynamic modeling is aimed at estimating the kinematic field (i.e., water levels and currents) responsible for the plume dispersion into the computational domain. The system of governing equations is rather complex and solved by numerical models with a high computational cost. This allows the study of very small spatial domains and for short-duration time windows. To overcome this limitation some simplifications are needed. These simplifications modify the governing equations (and therefore the processes that they are able to reproduce) to allow the analysis of larger areas and for longer time windows. In order to simplify the equations, it is important to identify the crucial key factors forcing the hydrodynamics. Just as an example, wave action plays a key role in the re-suspension and dispersion of sediments in relatively shallow water, while it can be intended as a secondary factor in deep water, where stratified phenomena must be taken into account instead. Indeed, waves and currents interact and influence each other (wave-current interaction). The presence of wave motion generates alterations in the hydrodynamic field that are almost negligible offshore, but may become significant in coastal areas. Even in transitional environments, usually characterized by shallow depths and mainly influenced by tidal oscillations, the action of wind waves produces hydrodynamic effects (and consequently transport phenomena due to interaction with the seabed) that are often not negligible. In turn, also the currents field can generate variations on the wave field (i.e., refraction). This phenomenon may become of great importance in areas such as transition environments characterized by the presence of river mouths or coastal areas characterized by the presence of intense local currents (e.g., rip currents, [42]).

Based on the selected driving forces, short wave propagation and long waves effects may be solved within either a coupled or uncoupled approach. Based on the importance of flow stratification, either two- (2DH), three- (3D), quasi-three-dimensional (Q3D) or multilayer models have to be considered. Table 2 synthesizes the applicability of the considered model types for a series of relevant cases within the frame of the mathematical modeling of physical effects induced by marine sediments handling works.

When wave propagation is addressed as a main driving force, the coupled approach aims at describing wave propagation by obtaining a detailed description of its time and spatial propagation. On the other hand, the coupling may be carried out by using the numerical results obtained by a wave propagation model as the forcing term of a hydrodynamic model able to give currents and water levels on a time scale longer than the short-waves period (and vice versa when the effects of currents on the wave propagation have to be considered).

3D numerical models are based on the resolutions of approximated equations solved in the three-dimensional space. The approximations (e.g., Reynolds Averaged Navier Stokes (RANS), large eddy simulation (LES)) are needed to make the numerical models usable within the frame of reasonably large domains. Nevertheless, they are characterized by large computational costs and then they are appropriate only when extremely detailed studies are needed. Examples of these models are NEMO (e.g., [43]), MOHID (e.g., [44]), ADCIRC (e.g., [45]), MIKE3 (e.g., [46]).

On the other hand, 2DH, quasi-3D (Q3D), and multi-layer models are based on equations integrated along the vertical direction. The use of 2DH models is appropriate when dealing with marine-coastal environments in which the vertical dimension of the domain, i.e., the water depth, is significantly smaller than the horizontal dimension (e.g., coastal and transition areas). However, it is necessary to pay attention to the applications for which the effects of vertical processes are important, such as stratified flows (e.g., river mouths with fresh water inlet in a salty environment) or wind driven circulation that can be characterized by high variations of the current profiles along the vertical direction. In such cases, it is possible to use models that, although not strictly three-dimensional, maintain information on the vertical variability of the quantities of interest (e.g., [47]). One approach is to hypothesize a given structure of the variability of quantities along the depth (Q3D models). Alternatively, it is possible to use several layers to integrate the governing equations by taking into account the flow stratification (multi-layer models). Examples of such a kind of models are SHORECIRC (e.g., [48]), DELFT3D-FLOW (e.g., [49]), MIKE21 (e.g., [50]), SHYFEM (e.g., [51]), POM (e.g., [52]), ROMS (e.g., [53]), SWASH (e.g., [54]), XBeach (e.g., [55]).

Table 2. Applicability of model type for a series of relevant cases, when model type as well as computational costs are accounted for. (++) suitable (even considering computational load with respect to expected results); (+): possible; (o): not completely suitable, hence the results may be affected by the model formulation; (-): not suitable, hence the results are strongly affected by the model formulation.

Case	Model Type	
	3D, Q3D, Multilayer	2DH
Shallow water dredging	(+)	(++)
Intermediate to deep water dredging	(++)	(-)
Dredging with re-suspension localized at the bottom	(++)	(-)
Dredging with homogeneous (along the water column) re-suspension	(+)	(++)
Disposal in coastal areas	(+)	(++)
Disposal in semi-enclosed basins with negligible flow stratification	(+)	(++)
Disposal in semi-enclosed basins with relevant wind action	(++)	(+)
Disposal in transitional areas	(++)	(o)
Disposal in transitional areas with significant stratification	(++)	(-)
Disposal in offshore areas	(++)	(o)

It has to be underlined that the hydrodynamic studies, i.e., the estimate of water levels and currents, need to take into account several driving forces in the computational domain and at the boundaries. The former, with different relevance depending on the area of application of the analysis (coastal and transitional areas, semi-closed basins, offshore areas), is made up of: wind and wave action, tidal oscillations, inlets characterized by different densities (e.g., river mouths or industrial discharges) for which it is necessary to take into account the buoyancy effects. The latter, on the other hand, consists of large-scale forcing, such as tidal induced currents and basin oscillations (e.g., wind setup, seiches).

The model must also take into account the physical processes related to the interaction of hydrodynamics with the boundaries of the area of interest (e.g., the sea bottom, the coastline and the open boundaries) as well as any elements placed within the calculation domain (e.g., coastal defenses, intertidal morphological structures in lagoon environments, bars or shafts in mouth areas, offshore structures if detectable by the resolution used in the model).

6.2. Sediment Transport and Deposition Modeling

Models for transport phenomena (dispersion, diffusion, and deposition) require the knowledge of the hydrodynamic field and the characteristics of the source term in order to produce reliable estimates of the spatial and temporal variability of suspended sediments (and of any associated contamination).

Numerical models for transport phenomena of suspended sediments are mainly distinguished in Eulerian and Lagrangian models on the basis of the selected approach to define the governing equation.

The Eulerian approach follows a formulation based on the description of the sediment concentration point by point, as given in Section 5 by Equation (4) in the special case of a two-dimensional approach. The resolution of the advection–diffusion equation allows for evaluating the space–time evolution of the SSC as a function of the hydrodynamic field and of the specific features of the source term. Similarly to hydrodynamic models, the governing equations can be simplified by averaging on small temporal or spatial scales (RANS and LES) by introducing parameters that represent the turbulence.

The Lagrangian method is based on a formulation that follows the spatial and temporal evolution of the position of individual particles, each representing a portion of the sediment plume. The main peculiarity of the mathematical formulation is that the effect of turbulence is represented by a stochastic formulation modeled by the random vector $\vec{d}_h$ (random walk models). As an example, the two-dimensional governing equation in the finite difference framework provided in [5,56] reads as follows:

$$\vec{r}(t+\delta t) = \vec{r}(t) + \delta t \left(\vec{v} + \sqrt{\frac{6k_h}{\delta t}} \vec{d}_h \right), \quad (5)$$

where $\vec{r}$ is the position vector of a specific individual particle, δt is the time step, $\vec{v}$ is the (horizontal) current field, k_h is the horizontal eddy diffusivity, and $\vec{d}_h$ is a vector with dimensionless components uniformly distributed in the range $[-1, +1]$. As an example, Figure 6 shows the particles dispersion due to the nearshore disposal during a beach nourishment intervention estimated by means of a random walk model.

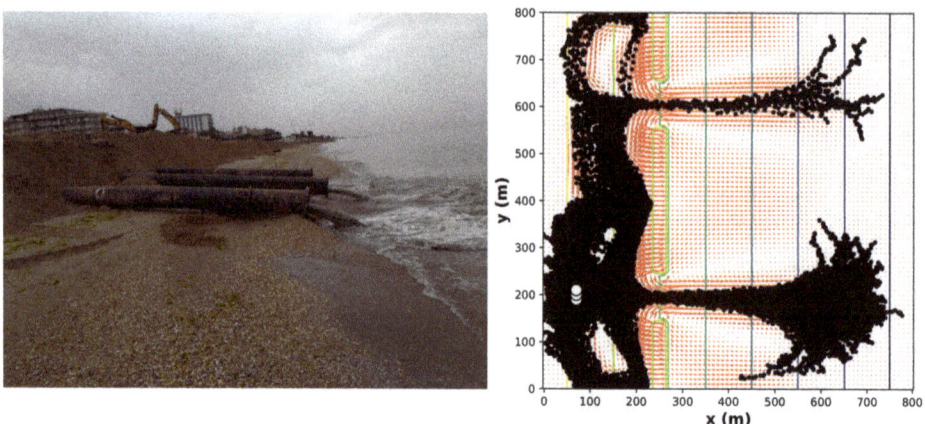

Figure 6. Typical results of a random walk model. The plot (**right**) refers to the dispersion of fine sediments due to nourishment (**left**) projects at a coastal defense cell when submerged breakwaters are present. Contour lines refer to the bathymetric configuration, arrows to the 2DH nearshore circulation forced by a sea state propagating along the x-direction, white circles indicate the re-suspension sources, black dots refer to the instantaneous location of passive tracers.

The use of Equation (5) is based on the hypothesis that the sediment is a passive tracer, i.e., it does not alter hydrodynamics, but is simply advected by the current field and progressively dispersed in the water column. The higher the sediment concentration, the lower the validity of this hypothesis, since the rheological behavior of the sediment-water mixture varies. As a consequence, this approximation is likely to be more acceptable in the far field than close to the sediment release source. The use of this hypothesis makes it possible to describe the sediment diffusion and transport process, decoupled from the hydrodynamic model. Alternatively, this aspect can be taken into consideration by altering the local value of the fluid density (also dependent on temperature and salinity). Considering that density also affects the hydrodynamic equations, it is then necessary to solve in a coupled way the two systems of equations (hydrodynamics and transport/diffusion). Many numerical models for hydrodynamics simulation include specific modules (Eulerian and/or Lagrangian) for sediment transport (e.g., [44,57,58]).

In order to improve the accuracy of the solutions, it is possible to consider different granulometric classes. In this case it is necessary to solve the equations separately for each class. In particular, this approach is useful to separate and better reproduce the dynamics of the finest fraction of sediment that undergoes transport processes in larger areas.

As far as DEP is concerned, there are many formulations available in the literature (e.g., [59–64]). For the deposition of non-cohesive sediments, it is possible to refer to the formulation proposed by Stokes, based on the assumption that the flow is in a viscous regime. However, when dealing with cohesive sediment it tends to underestimate deposition (and consequently to overestimate SSC). Therefore, in some cases, it is necessary to resort to formulations that take into account the presence of cohesive sediment (e.g., [65]), which can generate floccules for the attraction between particles that causes aggregation (e.g., [66–68]). Flocculation influences not only the effective diameter of the settling particles, but also the density, since floccules have a lower density than sediment particles with the same diameter [69].

Re-suspension of the sediments is an intensively studied problem but is still of interest (e.g., [70]). It is important to underline the differences in the re-suspension process as a function of the sediment characteristics. In fact, the size and density of the particles are the main factors influencing the re-suspension of non-cohesive sediments. Whereas, cohesive sediments, depending on the composition and the cohesion levels, can be grouped in two types: those that tend to aggregate into floccules when re-suspending and those whose re-suspension occurs as a muddy mixture [68]. Furthermore, cohesive and non-cohesive sediments are generally characterized by different consolidation processes. Non-cohesive sediments tend to consolidate rapidly and form a layer characterized by constant erodibility at the same depths. Cohesive sediments, on the contrary, tend to consolidate slowly and form cohesive base layers characterized by variable erodibility over time and depth. Re-suspension of cohesive sediments is mostly studied in the case of unidirectional or slowly variable currents (e.g., tidal currents), although the action of surface waves sometimes plays a significant role. In particular, the fluctuation of pressure values induced by the waves propagation can weaken and fluidize the sediment at the bottom [71,72]. The erodibility can also vary in relation to other physical, chemical and biological factors, such as the mineralogical composition, the presence of interstitial water and the pH, the ionic composition, the quantity and the type of organic matter in the different types of sediment (e.g., [68]).

Biological activity can also cause a temporal and spatial variability of the sediment erodibility (e.g., [73]). Re-suspension formulations are generally based on the comparison between the tangential stress (on the bottom) due to the hydrodynamics and a critical value of the tangential tension beyond which the sediment is re-suspended. This critical value is related to the geotechnical characteristics of the sediment [74,75] and is often assessed on an empirical basis [69].

7. Data Analysis and Representation

Past research works (e.g., [14,21,22,24,26,47,76]) show a lack of tools able to synthesize numerical results for supporting decision-makers in different design and environmental conditions. Maps showing the predicted (e.g., maximum and mean) SSC at different water depths and DEP, as well as time series at different key sites, are recommended to support planning and environmental approval. However, uniform criteria for the analysis and representation of numerical results obtained within preliminary modeling phase and detailed modeling phase have to be defined consistently with the characteristics of the modeling objectives. Indeed, they have to be defined based on the main physical processes identified as of primary interest for the considered environmental context, operational phase and environmental critical issues (if any) in the neighboring of the intervention site. Then, they can be useful also to select modeling scenarios (see Section 3) suitable to assess the fate and transport of the handled sediments with sufficient accuracy for the purpose of impact assessment.

An integrated, flexible and replicable methodological approach for synthesizing parameters related to water quality variations that arise from sediment handling activities is proposed herein starting from the extension of the environmental assessment method for dredging activity (Dr-EAM) methodology proposed by Feola et al. [26] to different environmental context (i.e., off-shore, near-shore and enclosed basin this paper deals with). These evaluations are needed for the assessment of the environmental impacts related to sediment handling projects and, in particular, for the evaluation of the severity of impacts on sensitive environmental receptors.

Based on past research works (e.g., [22,26]), it is recognized the importance of defining reference levels representative of the baseline variability of parameters of interest (e.g., SSC, DEP) before the handling operations or, during the activities, in reference areas potentially not affected by the handling works. A series of multiple reference levels with growing environmental criticality should be used to quantify the significance of the effects related to turbidity plumes during the project execution (e.g., [77]). These (single or multiple) reference levels must be established based on literature, site-specific monitoring and expert judgment depending on the project features (e.g., extension, duration, volume of handled sediments) and the expected interactions with the environmental critical issues (if any).

The source–path–receptor model can be used to represent the link between the sediment re-suspension source (intervention site) and the receptor (e.g., [18]). Although beyond the scope of this paper, it is important to stress that for a proper correlation between the significance of physical effects to the severity of possible impacts on the biological compartment, reference levels definition should also consider site-specific receptor tolerance limits (when they are available and/or they can be inferred from specific stress-response curves) to the expected water quality variation during execution. The severity of impacts is related to the presence of the expected and/or detected environmental issues, their location (with respect to sediment source and local currents), their nature and their ecological status (Figure 7).

The evaluation of the significance of effects must necessarily consider different aspects of the induced perturbations to the environmental effects, such as intensity, duration and frequency of events of SSC and DEP increase (e.g., [10,26,78–81]). The relationship between intensity, duration of perturbation and the related environmental effects on the specific receptor can be derived on the basis of site-specific data, on literature data or by expert judgment. When literature information or field data representative of the study area are not available, the reference levels can be defined using modeling studies in order to perform an analysis of the variability intervals of the parameters of interest. It is important to produce maps that summarize the modeling results [14]. Following the indications proposed by Feola et al. [26], a flexible, consistent and integrated methodological approach is presented in terms of standard and easily replicable techniques. The approach is suitable to support the identification and an easy assessment of the magnitude of potential effects in relation to intensity, duration and frequency of deviations from identified reference levels. In particular, it is useful to define a discrete number of check-points for extracting time series of output parameters throughout the whole period of simulation. Check-points have to be regularly distributed in the domain with a spatial scale chosen as a function of the spatial variability of the numerical results. For each check-point, time series can be extracted at different depths in the water column and at the seabed then analyzed and combined to derive suitable statistical parameters and indexes related to intensity, duration, and magnitude of exceedance of reference levels. Maps representing these parameters allow direct comparison of effects due to sediment handling works activity at progressive distances from the re-suspension zone. If the selected parameter is of hydrodynamic type, it will be possible to identify, for each scenario on both a seasonal and annual basis, zones with a different agitation level, as it will be possible to represent the spatial variability of the dispersion and deposition of the turbidity plume as SSC in water column and DEP at the bottom. To account for the combined effect of different parameters (e.g., duration and intensity), that cannot describe the significance of the exceedance of the reference level if separately considered, different methodological approaches can be used.

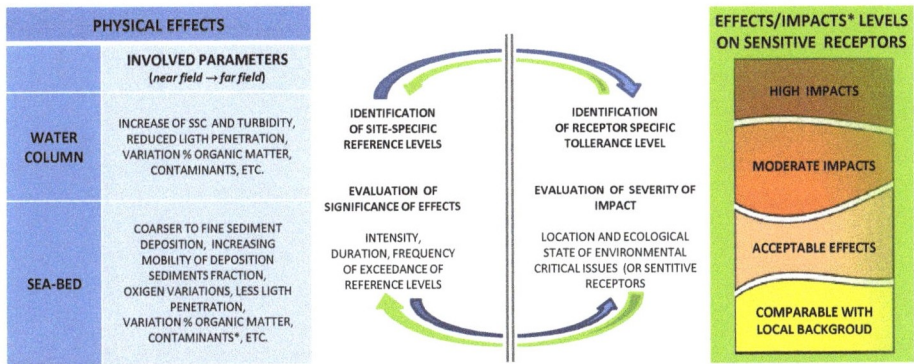

Figure 7. Scheme of the interactions between the significant physical effects related to the exceedance of reference levels (RLs) for SSC and sediment deposition rates (DEP) parameters and the severity of impact related to tolerance levels defined as a function of the status of sensitive receptors (if any).

A first approach for the definition of the significance of physical effects involves the use of a series of reference levels, the exceedance of which leads to the identification of intensities and durations. As an example, Figure 8 shows some indicative reference levels for intensity (SSC_{RL}) and duration intervals (T_{max_RL}), i.e., the maximum duration of time windows during which SSC exceeds the specific SSC_{RL}. The significance of the environmental effects is then defined in terms of a combination of SSC_{RL} and T_{max_RL}. Of course, the same method may be performed by changing the reference levels as a function of the specific receptor or by using other pairs of meaningful parameters (e.g., frequency of occurrence, [78]) on the basis of project-specific and/or site-specific and/or receptor-specific evaluations. In particular, synthetic maps are defined for each reference level in terms of intensity (e.g., SSC_{RL} = 10, 20, 50 mg/L in the example shown in Figure 8) storing at the single control point the significance value of the effect associated with the maximum duration of uninterrupted persistence of SSC above the specific value. From the overlap of the maps, the maximum value of registered significance is obtained for each specific control point. Maps can be overlapped to the location of sensitive habitats and ecological receptors in order to relate the sediment plume dynamic with different targets.

A second approach involves the use of a single index. Feola et al. [26] proposed to use the SSC number (SSC_{num}; mg s/L, e.g., [82]) that gives integral information about intensity, duration and frequency of exceedance of reference level. Basically, it is defined, for each simulation scenario (*i*), as the sum of the products of the mean intensity above reference level ($SSC_{mean\_RL,i}$) and the related duration (t_j, $j = 1 \ldots M_i$, with M_i the number of the considered events). Then, it reads (e.g., [26,82,83]):

$$SSC_{num,i} = \sum_{j=1}^{M_i} SSC_{mean\_RL,i} t_j \qquad (6)$$

where $SSC_{num,i}$ is the SSC number related to the specific *i*-th scenario. Maps of this integrated index can be then evaluated by analyzing the time series for each control point and for different values of the reference level.

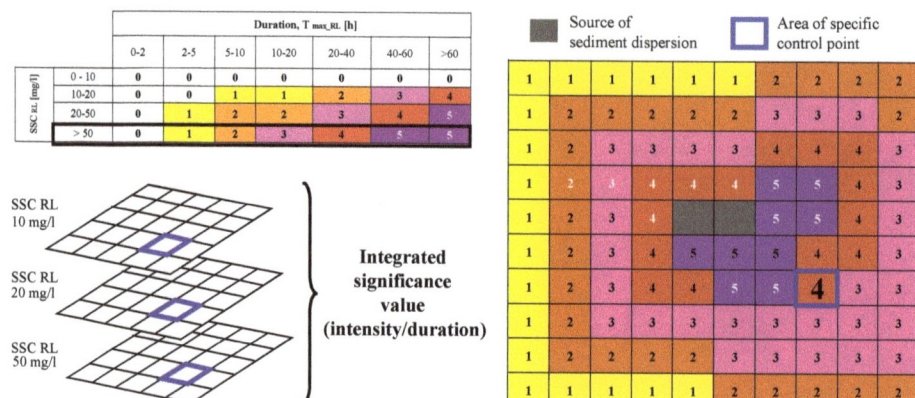

Figure 8. Example of maps of the significance of effects (based on intensity and duration) related to events of exceedance of reference levels (RLs). Significance classes are defined evaluating intensity and duration of exceedance of reference levels for increasing SSC (SSC_{RL} = 10, 20, 50 mg/L). Final significance level is the integrated result obtained by maps overlapping (right map).

Further useful analysis should be suitable to quantify the spatial and temporal variability of the effects associated with the dispersion of the turbidity plumes as a function of the distance from the sediment source. For these purposes semi-variograms can be used (e.g., [84]). Basically, the semi-variogram is defined as half of the averaged squared difference of the parameter at hand (SSC in this case) between points located at different distances. Then, the analysis of the semi-variogram allows the direct measurement of the spatial scale of the transport phenomena resulting from the generation of the turbidity plume and can be used to quantitatively compare the extent of the areas affected by the sediment handling activities (influence zone) related to different scenarios of simulation. The use of the semi-variogram provides the estimate of the variance (alteration with respect to the undisturbed value) of the parameter at hand modeled as a stochastic variable, and the estimate of the physical intensity of the alterations with respect to the undisturbed value.

8. The Role of Monitoring

8.1. Modeling and Monitoring Feedback System

Modeling–monitoring interactions are often recommended in environmental impact assessment procedures (and other regulatory frameworks) for assessing the compliance of selected operational criteria with the established environmental requirements. Basically, the selection of the modeling accuracy, and of the type of data to be collected as well, heavily depends on the general requirements of the various monitoring phases (before, during and after execution monitoring, e.g., [18]), and on the short- and long-term effects to be verified. Different types of data must be collected for determining the dynamics and the composition of turbidity plumes. The most common parameters needed to validate models are: sedimentological, meteo–climatic, hydrodynamic, water quality, topo–bathymetric and descriptive (e.g., coastline features, the presence of infrastructures or specific land-uses) data. The objective of measuring physical parameters not directly related to water quality (e.g., currents, waves, water elevations) is to provide information on how long a plume can remain in a particular area and on the time required for its dispersion to adjacent waters, as well as considering factors that may increase turbulence in the water column causing additional turbidity and preventing sedimentation.

In order to optimize a modeling–monitoring feedback system, typical environmental questions to be answered in the early preliminary planning phases are: (i) what types of sediment spill sources could be expected/distinguished (e.g., single point-spill event, continuous point-spill over a certain period); (ii) whether suspended sediments will leave the dredge- or dump-site; (iii) where the material will go and how much material will remain in the water column after a certain time. The most used parameter to characterize sediment plumes is turbidity, calibrated with in situ total suspended solids measures (TSS), defined as the total mass of material in a given volume of water, in mg/L. Nonetheless, establishing a reliable relationship between TSS and turbidity is not always possible because of the variation in characteristics of the suspended material. For defining turbidity values three aspects are usually considered: (i) turbidity level in the dredging area; (ii) the horizontal dispersion of the sediment cloud (for different hydrodynamics conditions); (iii) the settling time of the sediment cloud after cessation of operations. According to Pennekamp et al. [32], monitoring results allow the evaluations of the depth-averaged background concentration, of the characteristic increase of depth-averaged concentration at different distance from dredging/disposal activity, of the decay time of the re-suspended sediment after the execution of handling operations after which the turbidity return to background values, of the source term. In addition, chemical-physical parameters (temperature, salinity, conductivity and density conditions) are important to identify when sediment plumes significantly differ from the surrounding water. Dissolved oxygen and pH are commonly measured as indicators of water quality and of potential impact on biological resources (e.g., re-suspension of anoxic sediments may lower dissolved oxygen concentrations in the water column).

Fixed stations are required for comprehensive and regular monitoring over time. In fact, continuous time-series (single point or profiler) provide valuable information on the temporal variability of the monitoring variables along the water column. In particular, fixed stations allow collecting the background conditions during different environmental conditions before the execution of the works and to verify the selected reference levels during their execution.

During the execution phase, both fixed and mobile monitoring stations are required. Mobile stations (e.g., samplings from a vessel) are required when measurements at various locations over short-periods of time are needed, to one or more water depths, and to track the near-field plume through the water column. These types of measurements allows us to follow any change of the operational techniques that could influence sediment spill concentrations. Sampling time can be significantly increased depending both on site conditions (e.g., water depth and rate at which hydrodynamic conditions can vary) and on the purpose of the monitoring project phases.

The selection of the monitoring tools (i.e., fixed platforms, vessels, or towed vertical profilers) and of the sampling techniques is important to maximize the usefulness of the modeling–monitoring feedback system within the different phases of the project. Thus, understanding the advantages and limitations of the various available sampling techniques is important to determine the most cost-effective approach for sediment plumes monitoring. In general, using multiple instruments on the same platform reduces sampling time and provides synoptic measurements of the parameters being measured.

Based on the results of the monitoring and modeling analysis, it is possible to deepen the understanding of the system and its responses to pressures induced by changes on the involved environmental variables (chemical-physical and biological). Then it is possible to modify the design and monitoring choices. Mathematical models allow hydrodynamic and sediment transport evaluations (in time and space) for different selected spill scenarios, supporting the optimization of both work plans and environmental monitoring programs in the different project phases taking into account operational and environmental aspects. Monitoring data, on the other hand, are crucial to define input for near-field and far-field models, as well as for their calibration and validation and to verify the reliability of the modeling simplifications and results. For efficient management of sediment handling works, the modeling–monitoring feedback system is recommended herein as part of the proposed integrated modeling approach. The main relationships between modeling and monitoring activities and the main details on various deployment platforms for data collection (fixed platforms, vessels, or towed vertical profilers) at different stages of project design are highlighted in the followings.

Figure 9 shows the main interactions within the modeling–monitoring feedback system that should be carried out to verify the feasibility and the environmental compatibility of interventions in various design, execution and monitoring phases (i.e., before, during and after execution). In the preliminary design phase (i.e., before works execution), the modeling–monitoring feedback system serves as a supporting tool for the approval of work plans and for designing of suitable monitoring programs. In this context, the feedback between preliminary modeling spill scenarios and baseline-monitoring allows the selection of background conditions not related to the works execution. In particular, the determination of statistically reliable reference levels for the selected variables (e.g., SSC, DEP) will allow, during execution, to analyze monitoring and modeling results and to evaluate whether mitigation actions should be taken. Indeed, in the early stages of monitoring planning, site-specific information on types, distances and status of any sensitive objectives and receptors is needed for relating the significance of effects in terms of physical changes to the severity of impacts on critical targets (see Section 7).

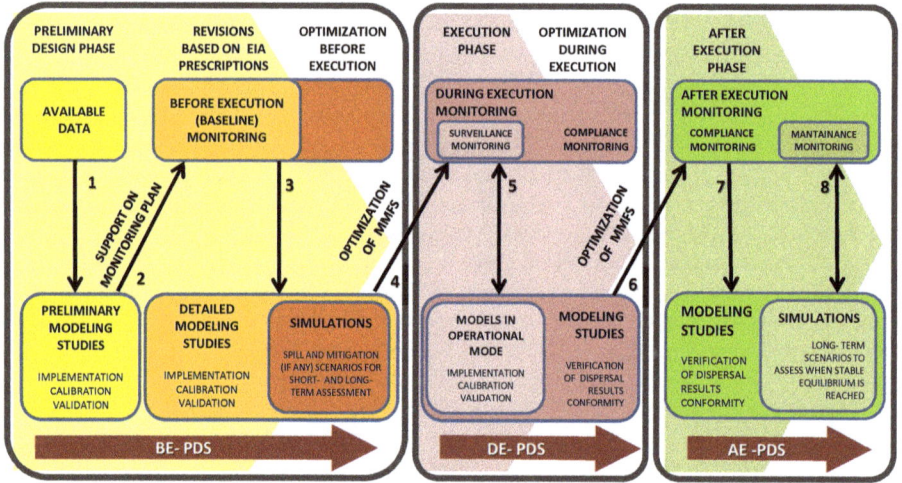

Figure 9. Scheme of the modeling–monitoring feedback system in the different phases of design, execution and management of handling operations. In the scheme, MMFS stands for modeling–monitoring feedback system; BE-BDS, DE-PDS and AE-PDS for project data sheets (PDS) before execution, during execution, and after execution, respectively; EIA for environmental impact assessment.

In fact, during and after sediment handling works, the modeling–monitoring feedback system is useful to verify (in the short-term) the fulfillment of the selected operational criteria and (in the short- and long-term) the compliance with the requirements of environmental protection mechanisms including legislation, contractor conditions and sustainability protocols [18]. In particular, changes of selected variables (e.g., SSC) can be compared with the selected (single or multiple) site-specific reference levels for water quality. For the short-term assessment, the surveillance monitoring is performed in the execution phase, trough the combined use of fixed and mobile (on-vessel) monitoring stations (see VBKO [85] and Aarninkhof et al. [86] for more details). This provides extensive sediment flux data useful for early warning to ensure that the amount of sediment re-suspension and dispersion is kept below the site-specific reference levels. Moreover, field data are crucial to validate the models to reduce the modeling uncertainties (i.e., the estimation of source terms). In addition, increasing knowledge on operational factors used to perform the sediment handling operations (e.g., more details on time schedule, production rate and type of dredges) should be considered for the set-up of more detailed modeling studies and for periodic reviewing of monitoring programs [17].

For interventions of considerable extension or in presence of very sensitive environmental critical issues (e.g., handling of pollutant sediments), the implementation of models in operational mode is useful to handle (mitigate or prevent) critical conditions that may occur during works execution (e.g., time windows of adverse weather and sea conditions, distribution of sediment concentration and sedimentation rates caused by natural or anthropogenic actions). In particular, the use of models in operational mode is recommended, as support to contractors and controlling authorities to promptly adopt proper alert procedures (e.g., interruption or modification of operations, implementations of mitigation measures) selected within a short term operation plan (STOP) aimed at ensuring that key parameters remain below specified alert levels (in term of both intensity and duration of exceedance), when these are forecast in one or more target points.

For the long-term assessment, a comprehensive and regular monitoring must be performed by means of fixed stations, including both the area involved by dispersal of re-suspended or spilled sediments and one or more periodic control points located in undisturbed areas (identified in advance trough the numerical modeling activities) and near environmental sensitive areas (if present). In this case, long-term scenarios should be implemented to forecast long-term effects and then verified through field measurements after the completion of the sediment handling operations. In particular, for a proper management plan, after works execution, monitoring should be performed until undisturbed conditions or a new stable equilibrium of the marine ecosystem (based on environmental considerations and criteria provided by controlling authorities) are achieved.

8.2. Management of Monitoring Data and Information Flow

According to the Adaptive Management approach (e.g., [7,17,87]), a sharing process between the contractor and the authority regarding the modeling–monitoring feedback system (to be foreseen before, during and after the conclusion of detailed studies) is desirable. The sharing process should include standard decision-making procedures and should be functional to optimize the work plan, the mitigation procedures (such as, modifications of dredging schedules, decrease of spill and overflow using special return pipes, closed grabs or clamshells, silt curtains or screens around dredgers) and the monitoring program (number, location and sampling frequency of the stations).

Moreover, within a modeling–monitoring feedback system, the implementation of an environmental information management system (EIMS) is encouraged to constantly enrich the available and usable data-set for a better application of the proposed integrated modeling approach (before, during and after each design and monitoring phases). In particular, project data sheets (PDSs) are promoted for a systematic collection and adequate dissemination of environmental (e.g., climatic an hydrodynamic conditions) and operational data (e.g., details on dredging equipment and techniques, production rate, work time schedules, type and operating mode of any mitigation measures) to be organized in a specific standardized, homogeneous and easily manageable format. This is in order to maximize the usefulness of monitoring data within the various design phases of the same project and to support the initial phases of future projects characterized by similar environmental and operating conditions. Indeed, the availability of data can be useful to increase the reliability of the modeling hypotheses, in particular for the estimation of source term. Information sheets can be considered as guides for data collection. In order to maximize the usefulness of PDSs their compilations should be performed with a frequency suitable to represent the natural background turbidity (e.g., for representative weather and sea conditions, vessel traffic). During the works, it is desirable to compile them also when operational parameters and site-specific environmental conditions change. In particular, the use of standard methodologies for the compilation of project data sheets before execution (BE-PDS), during execution (DE-PDS) and after execution (AE-PDS) phases (see Figure 9) will allow a good efficiency for calibration and validation processes and reliability of the obtained modeling results.

9. Concluding Remarks

This paper deals with the mathematical modeling needed to assess the physical effects induced by sediment handling operations in marine and coastal areas. In particular, it aims at:

- proposing an organic and comprehensive framework about the physical effects induced by sediments handling operations;
- detailing a broad-spectrum modeling approach intended to support contractors and controlling authorities in planning and managing sediment handling operations;
- illustrating an integrated, flexible and replicable methodological approach for synthesizing numerical results;
- highlighting the main features of the required modeling–monitoring feedback system.

The proposed integrated modeling approach for simulating sediment dispersion is intended as a flexible framework to estimate sediment dispersion due to marine sediment handling operations. It has been developed to assess the spatial and temporal variability of suspended sediment concentration and deposition rate by means of hydrodynamic, sediment source and transport models implementation. Different levels of accuracy are suggested for different project and operational phases based on the presence of environmentally sensitive critical issues (if any) and the classification of specific environmental contexts: coastal areas, semi-enclosed basins and offshore areas. In particular, paying attention to the feasibility of the modeling studies, it is proposed to perform a series of analyses with increasing details. Then, detailed (and computational onerous) simulations are suggested only if critical issues are likely to arise based on preliminary information and modeling phases. In order to guide the readers in all the steps of the proposed methodology, a further paper dealing with a series of case studies is in preparation.

One of the main uncertainties in the proposed integrated modeling approach implementation is related to the sediment source estimation. Indeed, site-specific data are required to obtain accurate estimate for release/sedimentation fluxes related to excavation, loads and dumping phases. Here the combined use of in situ data and numerical results is claimed to be powerful. Whereas the numerical results represent the variability of suspended sediment concentration at different time-scale far from the intervention site with acceptable reliability, in situ data are needed to gain insight on detailed aspects of the processes that influence its variability along the horizontal and vertical directions. Specific measurement and monitoring campaigns are among the challenges for giving more accurate model results. Then, the modeling–monitoring feedback system is proposed to be well suited as a framework to support the modeling practice, both with respect to the model and the data requirements. As part of the proposed modeling approach, it contributes to an integrated and application-oriented use of models and observations to monitor physical processes in different project phases (also in operational setting). Moreover, within a modeling–monitoring feedback system, the implementation of an environmental information management system and the compilation of project data sheets are promoted for a better application of the proposed integrated approach approach (before, during and after each design and monitoring phases). In particular, project data sheets compilation is encouraged to constantly enrich the available dataset and to maximize the usefulness of field data acquired during the various design phases of the project to be monitored and to support the initial phases of future projects characterized by similar environmental and operating conditions.

Author Contributions: Conceptualization, I.L., A.F., A.B., A.P., D.P. and M.D.R.; Data curation, I.L., A.F., A.B., A.P., D.P. and M.D.R.; Formal analysis, I.L., A.F., A.B., A.P., D.P. and M.D.R.; Investigation, I.L., A.F., A.B., A.P., D.P. and M.D.R.; Methodology, I.L., A.F., A.B., A.P., D.P. and M.D.R.; Software, I.L., A.F., A.B., A.P., D.P. and M.D.R.; Supervision, I.L.; Validation, I.L., A.F., A.B., A.P., D.P. and M.D.R.; Visualization, I.L., A.F., A.B., A.P., D.P. and M.D.R.; Writing—original draft, I.L., A.F., A.B., A.P., D.P. and M.D.R.; Writing—review & editing, I.L., A.F., A.B., A.P., D.P. and M.D.R.

Funding: This research received no external funding.

Acknowledgments: Massimo Gabellini is kindly acknowledged for his encouraging and precious suggestions. The authors wish to thank also Eng. Maurizio Ferla for his useful suggestions and for promoting the dissemination of the Italian Guidelines.

Conflicts of Interest: The authors declare no conflict of interest.

References

1. Ghosh, L.K.; Prasad, N.; Joshi, V.B.; Kunte, S.S. A study on siltation in access channel to a port. *Coast. Eng.* **2001**, *43*, 59–74. doi:10.1016/s0378-3839(01)00006-0. [CrossRef]
2. De Girolamo, P.; Romano, A.; Capozzi, F.; Franco, L.; Paganelli, M.; Di Risio, M.; Pasquali, D.; Sammarco, P.; Vink, N.; van Westendorp, P. Construction Aspects of the Civil Works for the Storm Surge Barrier at Chioggia Inlet–Venice. In *Coasts, Marine Structures and Breakwaters 2017*; ICE Publishing: London, UK, 2018.
3. Di Risio, M.; Lisi, I.; Beltrami, G.M.; De Girolamo, P. Physical modeling of the cross-shore short-term evolution of protected and unprotected beach nourishments. *Ocean Eng.* **2010**, *37*, 777–789. [CrossRef]
4. Saremi, S. Density-Driven Currents and Deposition of Fine Materials. Ph.D. Thesis, DTU Mechanical Engineering, Technical University of Denmark, Kongens Lyngby, Denmark, 2014.
5. Lisi, I.; Taramelli, A.; Di Risio, M.; Cappucci, S.; Gabellini, M. Flushing efficiency of Augusta harbour (Italy). *J. Coast. Res.* **2009**, *I*, 841–845.
6. Collins, M.A. *Dredging-Induced Near-Field Resuspended Sediment Concentrations and Source Strengths*; Technical Report; Southern Methodist University, School of Engineering and Applied Science: Dallas, TX, USA, 1995.
7. Eisma, D. *Dredging in Coastal Waters*; CRC Press: Boca Raton, FL, USA, 2005.
8. Becker, J.; van Eekelen, E.; van Wiechen, J.; de Lange, W.; Damsma, T.; Smolders, T.; van Koningsveld, M. Estimating source terms for far field dredge plume modelling. *J. Environ. Manag.* **2015**, *149*, 282–293. [CrossRef] [PubMed]
9. European Parliament and Council. Directive 2014/52/eu of the European Parliament and of the Council of 16 April 2014 amending Directive 2011/92/EU on the assessment of the effects of certain public and private projects on the environment. *Off. J. Eur. Union* **2014**, *124*, 1–18.
10. Clarke, D.; Engler, R.M.; Wilber, D. *Assessment of Potential Impacts of Dredging Operations Due to Sediment Resuspension*; Technical Report; Army Engineer Waterways Experiment Station: Vicksburg, MS, USA, 2000.
11. Erftemeijer, P.L.; Lewis III, R.R.R. Environmental impacts of dredging on seagrasses: A review. *Mar. Pollut. Bull.* **2006**, *52*, 1553–1572. [CrossRef]
12. Erftemeijer, P.L.; Riegl, B.; Hoeksema, B.W.; Todd, P.A. Environmental impacts of dredging and other sediment disturbances on corals: A review. *Mar. Pollut. Bull.* **2012**, *64*, 1737–1765. [CrossRef]
13. Lisi, I.; Di Risio, M.; De Girolamo, P.; Gabellini, M. Engineering tools for the estimation of dredging-induced sediment resuspension and coastal environmental management. In *Applied Studies of Coastal and Marine Environments*; InTech: London, UK, 2016.
14. GBRMPA. *Guidelines on the Use of Hydrodynamic Numerical Modelling for Dredging Projects in the Great Barrier Reef Marine Park August 2012*; Technical Report; Great Barrier Reef, Marine Park Authority: Townsville, Australia, 2012.
15. Lisi, I.; Feola, A.; Bruschi, A.; Di Risio, M.; Pedroncini, A.; Pasquali, D.; Romano, E. *La Modellistica Matematica Nella Valutazione Degli Aspetti Fisici Legati Alla Movimentazione dei Sedimenti in Aree Marino-Costiere*; Technical Report; ISPRA-Manuali e Linee Guida: Rome, Italy, 2017.
16. Savioli, J.; Magalhaes, M.; Pedersen, C.; Van Rijmenant, J.; Oliver, M.; Fen, C.; Rocha, C. Dredging-how can we manage it to minimise impacts. In Proceedings of the 7th International Conference on Asian and Pacific Coasts, Bali, Indonesia, 24–26 September 2013; Volume 6.
17. CEDA. *Integrating Adaptive Environmental Management into Dredging Projects*; Technical Report; Central Dredging Association: Delft, The Netherlands, 2015.
18. CEDA. *Environmental Monitoring Procedures*; Technical Report; Central Dredging Association: Delft, The Netherlands, 2015.
19. Becker, J. Dredge Plumes: Ecological Risk Assessment. Master's Thesis, Delft University of Technology, Delft, The Netherlands; National University of Singapore, Singapore, 2011.

20. Dupuits, E. Stochastic Effects of Dredge Plumes: Development and Application of a Risk-Based Approach to Assess Ecological Effects of Dredge Plumes on Sensitive Receivers. Master's Thesis, Delft University of Technology, Delft, The Netherlands, 2012.
21. Deltares. *Modelling of Sediment Dispersion Due to Maintenance Dredging. Lough Foyle, North Ireland*; Technical Report; Deltares: Delft, The Netherlands, 2009.
22. SKM. *Improved Dredge Material Management for the Great Barrier Reef Region*; Technical Report; Great Barrier Reef, Marine Park Authority: Townsville, Australia, 2013.
23. Johnson, B.H.; Andersen, E.; Isaji, T.; Teeter, A.M.; Clarke, D.G. *Description of the SSFATE Numerical Modeling System*; Technical Report; Army Engineer Waterways Experiment Station: Vicksburg, MS, USA, 2000.
24. Liu, J.T.; Chao, S.Y.; Hsu, R.T. Numerical modeling study of sediment dispersal by a river plume. *Cont. Shelf Res.* **2002**, *22*, 1745–1773. [CrossRef]
25. Jiang, J.; Fissel, D.B. Modeling Sediment Disposal in Inshore Waterways of British Columbia, Canada. In *Estuarine and Coastal Modeling (2011)*; American Society of Civil Engineers: Reston, VA, USA, 2012; pp. 392–414.
26. Feola, A.; Lisi, I.; Salmeri, A.; Venti, F.; Pedroncini, A.; Gabellini, M.; Romano, E. Platform of integrated tools to support environmental studies and management of dredging activities. *J. Environ. Manag.* **2016**, *166*, 357–373. [CrossRef]
27. European Parliament and Council. Directive 2008/56/EC of the European Parliament and of the Council of 17 June 2008 establishing a framework for community action in the field of marine environmental policy (Marine Strategy Framework Directive). *Off. J. Eur. Union* **2008**, *026*, 136–157.
28. Pasquali, D.; Bruno, M.; Celli, D.; Damiani, L.; Di Risio, M. A simplified hindcast method for the estimation of extreme storm surge events in semi-enclosed basins. *Appl. Ocean Res.* **2019**, *85*, 45–52. [CrossRef]
29. De Girolamo, P.; Di Risio, M.; Beltrami, G.; Bellotti, G.; Pasquali, D. The use of wave forecasts for maritime activities safety assessment. *Appl. Ocean Res.* **2017**, *62*, 18–26. [CrossRef]
30. John, S.; Challinor, S.; Simpson, M.; Burt, T.; Spearman, J. *Scoping the Assessment of Sediment Plumes Arising from Dredging*; Construction Industry Research & Information Association (CIRIA): London, UK, 2000.
31. Nakai, O. Turbidity generated by dredging projects. In *Management of Bottom Sediments Containing Toxic Substances, Proceedings of the 3rd U.S.-Japan Experts' Meeting, Easton, MD, USA, November 1977*; Report; United States Environmental Protection Agency, National Service Center for Environmental Publications: Cincinnati, OH, USA, 1978.
32. Pennekamp, J.G.; Epskamp, R.; Rosenbrand, W.; Mullie, A.; Wessel, G.; Arts, T.; Deibel, I. Turbidity caused by dredging: Viewed in perspective. *Terra et Aqua* **1996**, *64*, 10–17.
33. Hayes, D.F.; Crockett, T.R.; Ward, T.J.; Averett, D. Sediment resuspension during cutterhead dredging operations. *J. Waterw. Port Coast. Ocean Eng.* **2000**, *126*, 153–161. [CrossRef]
34. Hayes, D.; Wu, P.Y. Simple approach to TSS source strength estimates. In Proceedings of the WEDA XXI Conference, Houston, TX, USA, 25 June 2001; Volume 27.
35. Er, W.J.; Law, A.W.; Adams, E.E.; Zhao, B. Open-water disposal of barged sediments. *J. Waterw. Port Coast. Ocean Eng.* **2016**, *142*, 04016006. [CrossRef]
36. Henriksen, J.; Randall, R.; Socolofsky, S. Near-Field Resuspension Model for a Cutter Suction Dredge. *J. Waterw. Port Coast. Ocean Eng.* **2012**, *138*, 181–191. [CrossRef]
37. Roman-Sierra, J.; Navarro, M.; Muñoz-Perez, J.J.; Gomez-Pina, G. Turbidity and Other Effects Resulting from Trafalgar Sandbank Dredging and Palmar Beach Nourishment. *J. Waterw. Port Coast. Ocean Eng.* **2011**, *137*, 332–343. [CrossRef]
38. Hamin, E.; Abunnasr, Y.; Roman Dilthey, M.; Judge, P.; Kenney, M.; Kirshen, P.; Sheahan, T.; DeGroot, D.; Ryan, R.; McAdoo, B.; et al. Pathways to Coastal Resiliency: The Adaptive Gradients Framework. *Sustainability* **2018**, *10*, 2629. [CrossRef]
39. Di Risio, M.; Pasquali, D.; Lisi, I.; Romano, A.; Gabellini, M.; De Girolamo, P. An analytical model for preliminary assessment of dredging-induced sediment plume of far-field evolution for spatial non homogeneous and time varying resuspension sources. *Coast. Eng.* **2017**, *127*, 106–118. [CrossRef]
40. Shao, D.; Purnama, A.; Sun, T. Modeling the temporal evolution of dredging-induced turbidity in the far field. *J. Waterw. Port Coast. Ocean Eng.* **2015**, *141*, 04015001. [CrossRef]
41. Shao, D.; Gao, W.; Purnama, A.; Guo, J. Modeling dredging-induced turbidity plumes in the far field under oscillatory tidal currents. *J. Waterw. Port Coast. Ocean Eng.* **2016**, *143*, 06016007. [CrossRef]

42. Smith, G.G.; Weitz, N.; Soltau, C.; Viljoen, A.; Luger, S.; Maartens, L. Fate of fine sediment from dredger-based mining in a wave-dominated environment at Chameis Bay, Namibia. *J. Coast. Res.* **2008**, *24*, 232–247. [CrossRef]
43. Madec, G.; Delecluse, P.; Imbard, M.; Levy, C. *Ocean General Circulation Model Reference Manual*; LODYC: Paris, France, 1997; Volume 91.
44. Braunschweig, F.; Leitao, P.; Fernandes, L.; Pina, P.; Neves, R. The object-oriented design of the integrated water modelling system MOHID. In Proceedings of the XV International Conference on Computational Methods in Water Resources (CMWR XV), Chapel Hill, NC, USA, 13–17 June 2004; Elsevier: Chapel Hill, NC, USA, 2004; Volume 2, pp. 1079–1090.
45. Luettich, R.A., Jr.; Westerink, J.J.; Scheffner, N.W. *ADCIRC: An Advanced Three-Dimensional Circulation Model for Shelves, Coasts, and Estuaries. Report 1. Theory and Methodology of ADCIRC-2DDI and ADCIRC-3DL*; No. CERC-TR-DRP-92-6; Technical Report; Coastal Engineering Research Center: Vicksburg, MS, USA, 1992.
46. Danish Hydraulic Institute (DHI). *MIKE 21/MIKE 3 Flow Model FM: Hydrodynamic and Transport Module Scientific Documentation*; DHI: Copenhagen, Denmark, 2008.
47. Jiang, J. Investigation of key parameters for 3-D dredging plume model validation. In *Coasts and Ports 2011: Diverse and Developing, Proceedings of the 20th Australasian Coastal and Ocean Engineering Conference and the 13th Australasian Port and Harbour Conference, Perth, Australia, 28–30 September 2011*; Engineers Australia: Adelaide, Australia, 2011; p. 352.
48. Van Dongeren, A.; Sancho, F.; Svendsen, I.; Putrevu, U. SHORECIRC: A quasi 3-D nearshore model. *Coast. Eng.* **1994**, *1995*, 2741–2754.
49. Roelvink, J.; Van Banning, G. Design and development of DELFT3D and application to coastal morphodynamics. *Oceanogr. Lit. Rev.* **1995**, *11*, 925.
50. Warren, I.; Bach, H. MIKE 21: A modelling system for estuaries, coastal waters and seas. *Environ. Softw.* **1992**, *7*, 229–240. [CrossRef]
51. Umgiesser, G. *SHYFEM Finite Element Model for Coastal Seas, User Manual*; Georg Umgiesser: Venezia, Italy, 2012.
52. Mellor, G.L. *Users Guide for a Three Dimensional, Primitive Equation, Numerical Ocean Model*; Program in Atmospheric and Oceanic Sciences; Princeton University: Princeton, NJ, USA, 1998.
53. Shchepetkin, A.F.; McWilliams, J.C. The regional oceanic modeling system (ROMS): A split-explicit, free-surface, topography-following-coordinate oceanic model. *Ocean Model.* **2005**, *9*, 347–404. [CrossRef]
54. Zijlema, M.; Stelling, G.; Smit, P. SWASH: An operational public domain code for simulating wave fields and rapidly varied flows in coastal waters. *Coast. Eng.* **2011**, *58*, 992–1012. [CrossRef]
55. Roelvink, D.; Reniers, A.; Van Dongeren, A.; de Vries, J.V.T.; McCall, R.; Lescinski, J. Modelling storm impacts on beaches, dunes and barrier islands. *Coast. Eng.* **2009**, *56*, 1133–1152. [CrossRef]
56. Jouon, A.; Douillet, P.; Ouillon, S.; Fraunié, P. Calculations of hydrodynamic time parameters in a semi-opened coastal zone using a 3D hydrodynamic model. *Cont. Shelf Res.* **2006**, *26*, 1395–1415. [CrossRef]
57. Fachin, S.; Sancho, F. *M-Shorecirc: A New Morphodynamical Model*; International Coastal Symposium–ICS: Itapema, Brazil, 2004.
58. Warner, J.C.; Sherwood, C.R.; Signell, R.P.; Harris, C.K.; Arango, H.G. Development of a three-dimensional, regional, coupled wave, current, and sediment-transport model. *Comput. Geosci.* **2008**, *34*, 1284–1306. [CrossRef]
59. Özer, A. Simple equations to express settling column data. *J. Environ. Eng.* **1994**, *120*, 677–682. [CrossRef]
60. Ahrens, J.P. A fall-velocity equation. *J. Waterw. Port Coast. Ocean Eng.* **2000**, *126*, 99–102. [CrossRef]
61. Jiménez, J.A.; Madsen, O.S. A simple formula to estimate settling velocity of natural sediments. *J. Waterw. Port Coast. Ocean Eng.* **2003**, *129*, 70–78. [CrossRef]
62. Ferguson, R.; Church, M. A simple universal equation for grain settling velocity. *J. Sediment. Res.* **2004**, *74*, 933–937. [CrossRef]
63. Je, C.H.; Chang, S. Simple approach to estimate flocculent settling velocity in a dilute suspension. *Environ. Geol.* **2004**, *45*, 1002–1009. [CrossRef]
64. Mehta, A.J.; McAnally, W.H. Fine grained sediment transport. In *Sedimentation Engineering: Processes, Measurements, Modeling, and Practice*; Garcia, M., Ed.; ASCE: Reston, VA, USA, 2008; Chapter 4, pp. 253–306.
65. Soulsby, R.; Manning, A.; Spearman, J.; Whitehouse, R. Settling velocity and mass settling flux of flocculated estuarine sediments. *Mar. Geol.* **2013**, *339*, 1–12. [CrossRef]

66. Milburn, D.; Krishnappan, B. Modelling Erosion and Deposition of Cohesive Sediments from Hay River, Northwest Territories, Canada: Paper presented at the 13th Northern Res. Basins/Workshop (Saariselkä, Finland and Murmansk, Russia-Aug. 19-24 2001). *Hydrol. Res.* **2003**, *34*, 125–138. [CrossRef]
67. Je, C.H.; Hayes, D.F.; Kim, K.S. Simulation of resuspended sediments resulting from dredging operations by a numerical flocculent transport model. *Chemosphere* **2007**, *70*, 187–195. [CrossRef]
68. Winterwerp, J.C.; Van Kesteren, W.G. *Introduction to the Physics of Cohesive Sediment Dynamics in the Marine Environment*; Elsevier: Amsterdam, The Netherlands, 2004; Volume 56.
69. Sun, C.; Shimizu, K.; Symonds, G. Numerical modelling of dredge plumes: A review. *Report of Theme*, June 2016, p. 45.
70. Valipour, R.; Boegman, L.; Bouffard, D.; Rao, Y.R. Sediment resuspension mechanisms and their contributions to high-turbidity events in a large lake. *Limnol. Oceanogr.* **2017**, *62*, 1045–1065. [CrossRef]
71. Mehta, A.J. Interaction between fluid mud and water waves. In *Environmental Hydraulics*; Springer: Berlin/Heidelberg, Germany, 1996; pp. 153–187.
72. Celli, D.; Li, Y.; Ong, M.C.; Di Risio, M. The role of submerged berms on the momentary liquefaction around conventional rubble mound breakwaters. *Appl. Ocean Res.* **2019**, *85*, 1–11. [CrossRef]
73. Grabowski, R.C.; Droppo, I.G.; Wharton, G. Erodibility of cohesive sediment: The importance of sediment properties. *Earth-Sci. Rev.* **2011**, *105*, 101–120. [CrossRef]
74. Gularte, R.C.; Kelly, W.; Nacci, V. Erosion of cohesive sediments as a rate process. *Ocean Eng.* **1980**, *7*, 539–551. [CrossRef]
75. Parchure, T.M.; Mehta, A.J. Erosion of soft cohesive sediment deposits. *J. Hydraul. Eng.* **1985**, *111*, 1308–1326. [CrossRef]
76. IMDC. *Environmental Impact Assessment Windmill Farm Rentel, Numeric Modelling of Dredging Plume Dispersion*; Technical Report; International Marine & Dredging Consultants: Antwerp, Belgium, 2012.
77. Sofonia, J.J.; Unsworth, R.K.F. Development of water quality thresholds during dredging for the protection of benthic primary producer habitats. *J. Environ. Monit.* **2010**, *12*, 159–163. [CrossRef] [PubMed]
78. Wilber, D.H.; Clarke, D.G. Biological Effects of Suspended Sediments: A Review of Suspended Sediment Impacts on Fish and Shellfish with Relation to Dredging Activities in Estuaries. *N. Am. J. Fish. Manag.* **2001**, *21*, 855–875. doi:10.1577/1548-8675(2001)021<0855:beossa>2.0.co;2. [CrossRef]
79. Fraser, M.W.; Short, J.; Kendrick, G.; McLean, D.; Keesing, J.; Byrne, M.; Caley, M.J.; Clarke, D.; Davis, A.R.; Erftemeijer, P.L.A.; et al. Effects of dredging on critical ecological processes for marine invertebrates, seagrasses and macroalgae, and the potential for management with environmental windows using Western Australia as a case study. *Ecol. Indic.* **2017**, *78*, 229–242. doi:10.1016/j.ecolind.2017.03.026. [CrossRef]
80. Jones, R.; Bessell-Browne, P.; Fisher, R.; Klonowski, W.; Slivkoff, M. Assessing the impacts of sediments from dredging on corals. *Mar. Pollut. Bull.* **2016**, *102*, 9–29. doi:10.1016/j.marpolbul.2015.10.049. [CrossRef]
81. Fisher, R.; Walshe, T.; Bessell-Browne, P.; Jones, R. Accounting for environmental uncertainty in the management of dredging impacts using probabilistic dose-response relationships and thresholds. *J. Appl. Ecol.* **2018**, *55*, 415–425. doi:10.1111/1365-2664.12936. [CrossRef]
82. Erm, A.; Tarmo, S. The impact of fast ferry traffic on underwater optics and sediment resuspension. *Oceanologia* **2006**, *48*, 283–301.
83. Rapaglia, J.; Zaggia, L.; Ricklefs, K.; Gelinas, M.; Bokuniewicz, H. Characteristics of ships' depression waves and associated sediment resuspension in Venice Lagoon, Italy. *J. Mar. Syst.* **2011**, *85*, 45–56. [CrossRef]
84. Matheron, G. Principles of geostatistics. *Econ. Geol.* **1963**, *58*, 1246–1266. doi:10.2113/gsecongeo.58.8.1246. [CrossRef]
85. VBKO. *Protocol for the Field Measurements of Sediment Release from Dredgers*; Technical Report; VBKO: Surrey, UK, 2003.
86. Aarninkhof, S.; Rosenbrand, W.; Van Rhee, C.; Burt, T. The day after we stop dredging: A world without sediment plumes? *Terra et Aqua* **2008**, *110*, 15–24.
87. CEDA-IADC. *Dredging for Sustainable Infrastructure*; Central Dredging Association (CEDA) and International Association of Dredging Companies (IADC): Delft, The Netherland, 2018.

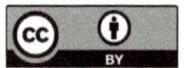

© 2019 by the authors. Licensee MDPI, Basel, Switzerland. This article is an open access article distributed under the terms and conditions of the Creative Commons Attribution (CC BY) license (http://creativecommons.org/licenses/by/4.0/).

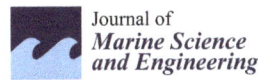

Article

Influence of Underwater Bar Location on Cross-Shore Sediment Transport in the Coastal Zone

Olga Kuznetsova [1,2,*] and Yana Saprykina [2]

[1] Zubov State Oceanographic Institute of Roshydromet, Russian Academy of Sciences, Moscow 119034, Russia
[2] Shirshov Institute of Oceanology, Russian Academy of Sciences, Moscow 117997, Russia; saprykina@ocean.ru
* Correspondence: olga.ku-ocean@yandex.ru; Tel.: +7-903-557-9035

Received: 31 December 2018; Accepted: 21 February 2019; Published: 26 February 2019

Abstract: The effect of the underwater bar position on a sandy beach profile was studied on a timescale of one storm, using the XBeach numerical model. The largest shoreline regress occurred in the first hour of storm. For the chosen wave regime an underwater profile close to the theoretical Dean's equilibrium profile is formed after 6 h. The position of the underwater bar affects the shoreline retreat rate. The lowest shore retreat occurs when the bar crest is located at a distance equal to 0.70–0.82 of the deep-water wavelength, corresponding to the period of the wave spectrum peak. The maximal shoreline retreat occurs when the bar is located at a distance that is close to a half wavelength. The shoreline recession depends on the heights of low-frequency waves. The smaller the mean wave period and the higher low-frequency waves' height near the coast, the smaller the retreat of the shoreline. The distance of seaward sediment transfer is directly proportional to the significant wave height near shore.

Keywords: coastal zone; storm deformations; underwater bar; XBeach; wave transformation; cross-shore sediment transport; equilibrium profile

1. Introduction

Hydrodynamic processes are important factors in coastal zone evolution. The off- and onshore relief of sandy beaches is deeply bound with the wave regime. The wave climate and its variations are main mechanisms of cross-shore sediment transport in the coastal zone; for instance, the formation and movement of underwater longshore bars, which are observed on many sandy coasts [1–3].

Around 10% of sea coasts have underwater bars [4]. The timescale of longshore bar formation and movement can vary from days to months [5]. According to laboratory experiments [3], under weak or moderate waves, the underwater bar moves shoreward until it joins the coast and disappears. Stronger waves switch the direction of the bar movement seaward. With changing wave conditions, the underwater bar can stay approximately at the same place and be considered stable [3].

Underwater bars are specific features of the bottom relief, so that they affect a wave transformation process within a coastal zone. As a result, the bars have influence on a cross-shore sediment transport and shoreline deformations. The wave transformation over barred profiles of sandy beaches and the corresponding morphodynamical features are a challenging and intensively studied topic [1–3,6].

Nevertheless, the role of underwater bar positioning in shoreline dynamics is still not obvious. From an engineering point of view, this issue is important for coastal defense, and it should be clarified [7]. Artificial underwater bars and reefs that imitate natural structures have become popular in coastal engineering [8]. Such constructions (breakwaters) are installed in order to decrease the wave load on the coast and reduce erosion. The decline of wave energy occurs due to breaking and shortening of the mean wave period by non-linear dispersive wave transformation over bars [9]. A similar effect is also detected in studies devoted to the impact of wave farms on nearshore wave conditions and coastal protection [10]. It is crucial to find an appropriate position and an optimal shape for artificial underwater structures, in order to obtain the maximum benefits. Thus, a detailed study of the influences of the bar position on wave transformation, the corresponding sediment transport in the coastal zone, and the rate of wave-induced shoreline erosion, is a very important scientific and coastal engineering task.

The goal of this work is to investigate the influence of the underwater bar position (off a non-tidal sea coast) on the transformation of waves above it, and on corresponding cross-shore sediment transport, on the timescale of a strong storm.

2. Materials and Methods

During the field experiments at the Shkorpilovtsy study site (Black Sea, Bulgaria) [11], we noticed the festoon-shaped features of the shoreline. Satellite images show that the onshore festoon-pattern is accomplished by crescent underwater bars (Figure 1). According to long-term observations [11,12], the bars migrate slightly, depending on variations in the wave conditions. The shoreline shape has inter-annual variations that are possibly associated with the features of the underwater bottom relief. This fact induced us to prove the idea that the location of the underwater bar defines the shape of shoreline to some extent.

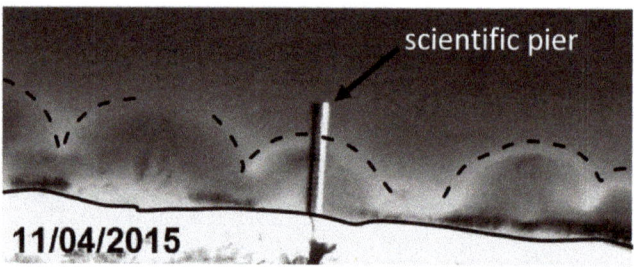

Figure 1. Satellite image of the crescent underwater bars at the Shkorpilovtsy study site (Image © 2017 Digital Globe). Dotted line: the crest of the bar; solid: the water's edge.

Numerical computation by using XBeach [13] has been chosen as a main tool, because this is a well-developed and popular open-source hydrodynamic and morphology modelling package [14,15]. The non-hydrostatic mode of XBeach, which we used for wave and bottom changes modelling, resolves short waves and provides an accurate reproduction of wave propagation in shallow water [16]. In contrast to stationary or surf-beat mode, the non-hydrostatic mode resolves the wave profile, and it does not require additional wave asymmetry correction.

Although the main goal of the research involves a purely numerical experiment, it is still important to set reasonable realistic boundary conditions. For this purpose, we used field observations (bathymetry and sediment properties) from the Shkorpilovtsy study site [17], as well as information about the wave climate in the north-western part of the Black Sea [18,19].

A numerical grid (1D) was built, based on a set of 12 cross-shore profiles, measured in a frame of the international field experiment "Shkorpilovtsy-2007". All of the observed profiles that were made along the beach had a bar that was located at different distances from shore. From the observed data, we obtained a characteristic shape of the bottom profile and the underwater bar.

The average bottom profile on the Shkorpilovtsy coast has no bar. It has a slope of 0.022, a slight increase of the slope in the upper part, and a small terrace at 2–3 m depth. This profile was considered to be used for modelling, and it was a basis for the creation of a set of barred profiles.

The characteristic shape of the underwater bar was superimposed with a mean profile at a different distance from the shoreline. Thus, five synthetic profiles were created with different bar positionings (Table 1, Figure 2).

Table 1. Parameters of the initial profiles.

Parameter	Profile					
	0	1	2	3	4	5
Depth over the bar crest, m	None	−3.07	−2.68	−2.38	−2.20	−2.08
Bar crest location (x-coordinate), m	None	714	730	748	762	784
Distance between shoreline and the bar crest (X), m (distance (X)/wave length (L))	None	141 (0.82)	125 (0.72)	107 (0.62)	93 (0.54)	73 (0.42)

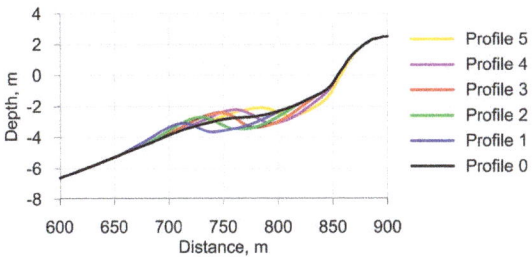

Figure 2. The cross-shore profiles used as the model bathymetry input.

The spatial resolution of the grid was set to 2 m, as calculated using Matlab Toolbox, which has been created and recommended specifically for this purpose, according to the XBeach developers. The Toolbox helps XBeach users to choose appropriate grid settings, taking into account the wave parameters and the relief characteristics. The Black Sea is a non-tidal sea, and so the initial water level was set at 0 m for all of the simulations.

The sediment on the Shkorpilovtsy beach are anisogamous quartz sands. More than 95% of the bottom sediments in the upper part of profile (till 2.5 m) are coarse-grained or medium. For the modelling, we used medium grain, with a diameter D50 (d50) of 0.2 mm.

The validation of XBeach, which has been made by developers and users, shows that this package can be successfully used in non-hydrostatic mode with the default settings [20]; however, some studies have shown that XBeach overestimates coastal erosion [21], which we also noticed from our analysis of the field data and the modelling results. For study site conditions, we tested XBeach with stationary and non-stationary (Joint North Sea Wave Project Spectrum - JONSWAP) wave inputs, and compare these with the synchronous observations carried out during field experiment <Skorpilovtsy-2007> (Figure 3). The results could be considered reasonable.

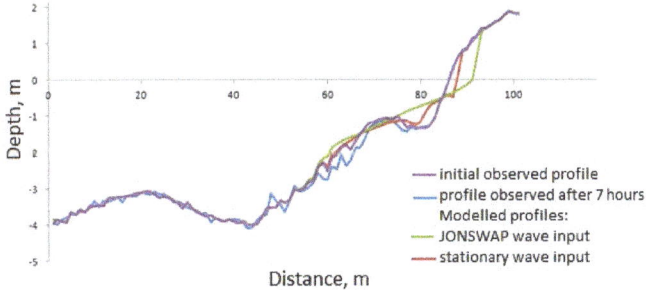

Figure 3. Results of the XBeach verification for the Shkorpilovtsy study site, for cases of 7 h wave action (significant wave height Hs = 0.9 m, and spectral peak period Tp = 7 s).

The goal of the research was to investigate the wave-bottom adjustment on the time scale of one storm. For this reason, we defined the wave input in accordance with typical storm conditions, presented in the wave climate descriptions of Black Sea [18,19]. The wave input was set at the sea boundary of the numerical grid (≈860 m from shore) in the form of JONSWAP wave spectra, with the following parameters: peak enhancement factor γ = 3.3, significant wave height Hs = 1.5 m, spectral peak period Tp = 10.5 s, wave energy-spreading angle δ = 2.5°. A storm with wave heights of 1.5 m was considered to be a dangerous hydrometeorological phenomenon in the Azov–Black Sea region [22]. A wave period of 10.5 s corresponded to extreme storms with return periods of 25 years [18]. The duration of a single storm event was set to 20 h, in accordance with the criteria developed for the Black region by Belberov [23], and for Atlantic coasts by Lozano [24], also taking into account the World Meteorological Organization recommendations for meteorological observations [25].

The modelling process was organized according to the following algorithm. In first hour of wave action, there was no morphology changes, but there was a wave output with very fine time resolution (5 Hz). Modelling was continued for another 20 h, with relief changes enabled. The output of the bathymetry was set every hour.

From the first step of the computation, we obtained free surface elevation data along the profile between the coordinates 620–820 m (see Figure 4). This part corresponded with depths of 2–6 m. The sampling frequency of the time series was 5 Hz. Chronograms were used for the calculation of the wave spectra, and for the following wave parameters [26]:

1. Significant wave height (in m), calculated as:

$$H_S = 4 \cdot \sqrt{m_0} \tag{1}$$

where:

$$m_0 = \int_0^\infty S(\omega) d\omega \tag{2}$$

and $S(\omega)$ are the spectra, ω is the angular frequency, with linear frequency filters: 0–0.05 Hz chosen to account for a significant wave height of low frequency range, including infragravity waves (H_{IGW}).

2. The mean wave period(s) is/are as follows:

$$T_{mean} = \frac{\int_0^\infty S(\omega) d\omega}{\int_0^\infty \omega \cdot S(\omega) d\omega} \tag{3}$$

3. The wave asymmetry coefficient (with asymmetry relative to the vertical axis):

$$As = \frac{\langle \zeta_H^3 \rangle}{\sigma^3} \tag{4}$$

where $\langle \rangle$ is the averaging operator, ζ are the free surface elevations, σ is the standard deviation of the free surface elevations, and ζ_H is the Hilbert transform.

4. The wave-skewness coefficient (relative to the horizontal axis):

$$Sk = \frac{\langle \zeta^3 \rangle}{\sigma^3} \tag{5}$$

From the second step of computation, we obtained the hourly data of the computed morphology changes for over 20 h of wave action. Based on a set of calculated profiles, the coastline retreat and the change in the underwater bottom relief were evaluated.

J. Mar. Sci. Eng. **2019**, *7*, 55

The parameters of the underwater bar for the initial profiles (input conditions) are shown in Table 1. The wave length was determined by the dispersion relation of the linear waves' theory for the spectral peak period.

3. Results

Figure 3 shows the underwater bottom profiles, both initially and the result of 20 h storm modelling. The resulting deformations of the underwater profile are presented in Table 2. The change in all of the beach profiles was characterized by erosion in the splash area, the transition of material seaward, and its accumulation at depths of more than 1 m. However, the activity of erosion and accumulation processes on profiles with different bar locations varied.

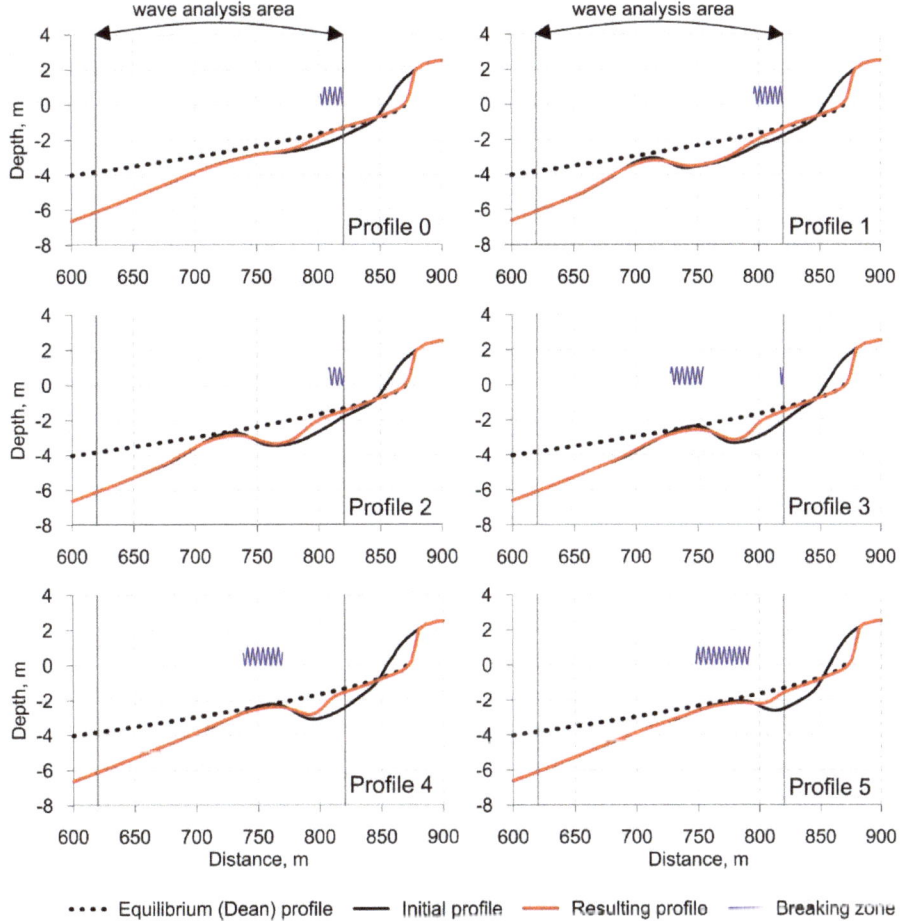

Figure 4. Initial and resulting profiles after 20 h of wave action (Hs = 1.5 m, Tp = 10.5 s), location of the breaking zone, and theoretical shape of the equilibrium profile calculated for a grain size of 0.2 mm.

Table 2. Main changes in model profiles after 20 h of wave action.

Parameter	Profile					
	0	1	2	3	4	5
Depth over the bar crest, m	None	−3.21	−2.86	−2.59	−2.37	−2.18
Distance between the shoreline and the bar crest (X), m (distance (X)/wavelength (L))	None	141 (0.82)	125 (0.72)	107 (0.62)	93 (0.54)	73 (0.42)
Shoreline regression (Sh), m	14.8	14.3	15.3	16.7	17.6	15.6
Average accretion layer, m	0.34	0.29	0.30	0.41	0.50	0.61
Distance of sediment transportation (x), m (Distance of sediment transportation (x) / Wavelength (L))	76 (0.44)	86 (0.50)	98 (0.57)	82 (0.48)	70 (0.41)	54 (0.31)

In general, if a bar is located closer to the coast and it has reduced depth above it, several patterns can be distinguished: the rate of shore erosion increases, the thickness of the sediment accumulation layer in the underwater part of the profile decreases, and the distance of sediment transfer to the sea grows (Table 2). However, the shoreline recession (Figure 5a) on the profile with the furthest bar position (0.82 from the wavelength) was substantially less than that of the profile where the bar was located closer to the shore (0.42 from the wavelength). The coastline degradation on the profile where the bar was positioned at 0.54 from the wavelength was maximum for all of the considered profiles. The seaward transfer distance of the sediment (Figure 5b) was maximal on the profile where the bar is positioned, at 0.82 (profile 1) from the wavelength. In all cases, there was no transport of sediments beyond the bar (Figure 4).

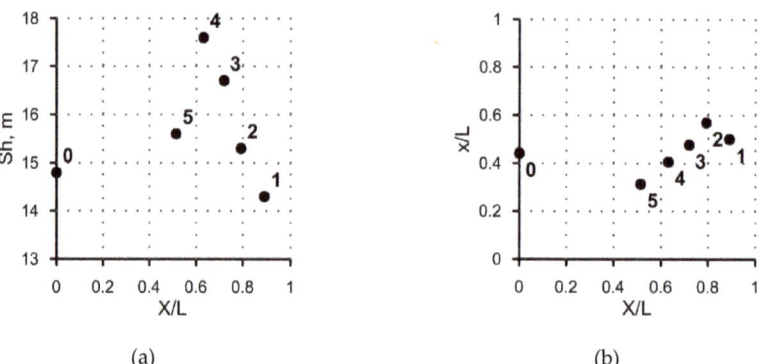

(a) (b)

Figure 5. (a) Shoreline regression (Sh, m) and (b) distance of seaward sediment transport, in terms of wavelength (x/L) independence of the initial bar location (X/L). X is the distance between the bar crest and the shoreline, x is the distance of the maximum amounts of sediments that are transported away from the shore, L is the wavelength calculated for deep-water conditions

Compared to the profile without a bar, the profile with the furthest bar location (the relative distance from the coast is 0.82 of wavelength) reduces the degree of shoreline degradation. The profile with the closest position to the bar (a relative distance from the coast of 0.42, or less than half the wavelength) worked best as a barrier against carrying the beach material seaward to depth. Compared with a barless control profile, an underwater bar at some relative distances from the coast could lead to an increase in coastline degradation.

Under the storm waves, slight deformations of bars also occurred (Figure 4): the reduction of its relative height, the deepening of the bar top (on profile 5), and a retreat of the bar crest (2–4 m) towards the sea (on profiles 1, 2, and 4). The bar shape changed with regard to its slope oriented towards the coast, which became less steep due to the filling of the bar trough. Such movements of the bar crest and the change in its asymmetry are generally consistent with the data of field observations [17].

The process of the retreat of the coastline and the transformation of the coastal zone relief occurs non-uniformly over time. Figure 6 shows the changes in the coastline retreat speed after 10 h of wave action, for profiles with maximum (4) and minimum (1) changes. The fastest shoreline retreat was observed during the first hour of the storm for all profiles: it varied from 4.5 to 6.5 m/h. Erosion activity slows down over time. After 6 h of wave action, the beach profile adapts to the specific waves occurring, and assumed a relatively equilibrium state. The shoreline regression rate became ≈0.5 m/h, and it remained approximately the same for all profiles.

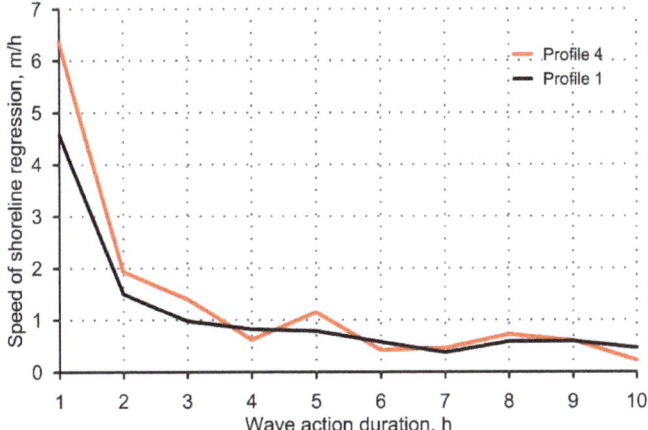

Figure 6. The speed of shoreline regression (m/h) variations during the numerical experiment that was run on profiles 1 (black) and 4 (red).

Regardless of the initial underwater relief, an underwater terrace was is formed on for all profiles (Figure 4), representing an equilibrium profile that was close to the theoretical classical Dean's profile proposed in [27]:

$$h = Ax^{2/3} \qquad (6)$$

where $A = 0.1$, calculated for a sediment grain size of 0.2 mm [26]. The formation of an underwater profile of similar shape with a terrace under the influence of uniform storm waves was also observed by us in the field experiment "Shkorpilovtsy 2007" [17].

Different degrees of coastline degradation during the first hour of the storm can be explained by differences in the transformation of the storm waves along the bottom profiles. Figure 7 shows the dependencies of the change in the coastline retreat, and the sediment seaward transfer distance on the relative change in the significant wave heights, as determined by the ratio of the corresponding values before and after the bar (with coordinates on model profiles 620 and 820 m). The significant wave height slightly decreases when the waves came nearer to the shore, but the decline was more strongly expressed in profiles 4 and 5, where the bar is located near the shore. On profiles 1–3, the significant wave height fall was less than in the profile without a bar. The distance of seaward sediment transport directly depends on the significant wave height: the greater the height, the further the material is transferred (Figure 7b). The relation between the shoreline regression and the change in significant wave height was not so clear (Figure 7a).

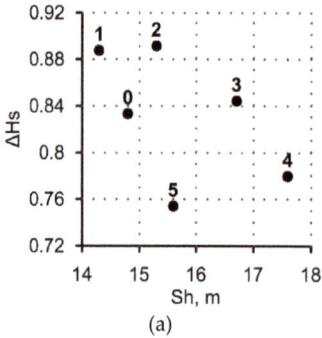 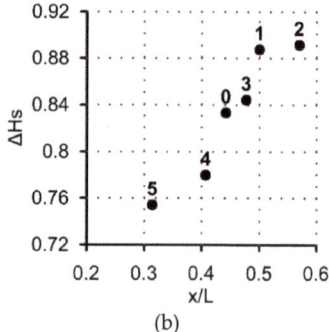

Figure 7. Dependence of (**a**) the shoreline retreat (Sh, m) and (**b**) the relative distance of seaward sediment transport (x/L) on the relative change in significant wave height (ΔHs, m) occurring during wave transformation over barred profile (620–820 m, see Figure 4). L is wave length calculated for deep water conditions, x is distance of maximal sediments transport away from the shore

The shoreline retreat is influenced more by the mean wave period than by wave height. Figure 8 depicts the relation between bottom deformations and relative change of mean wave period determined by the ratio of the corresponding values before and after the bar (coordinates on model profile 620 and 820 m). The smaller the change in the mean wave period, the smaller the degradation of the coastline (Figure 8a). Such a change of parameters occurred in profile 1, with a bar being located at a distance from the shoreline of 0.82 of a wavelength. There was no clear dependence of sediment transport on the mean period.

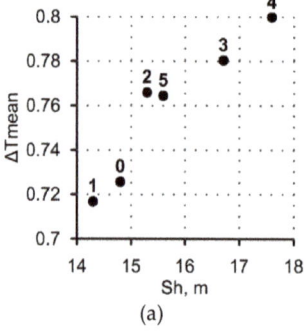 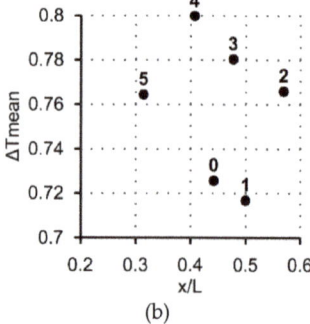

Figure 8. Dependence of (**a**) shoreline retreat (Sh, m) and (**b**) the relative distance of seaward sediment transport (x/L) on the relative change in the mean wave period (ΔTmean, s) occurring during wave transformation over a barred profile (620–820 m, see Figure 4). L is the wavelength calculated for deep-water conditions, and x is the distance of maximal sediment transportation away from the shore.

The modelling of profiles with five different bar locations shows that a growth of significant height in the low-frequency waves after passing a bar leads to a decline of coastline degradation (Figure 9a). This relation is close to linear, except for profile 5, where the change in the low-frequency wave height is the same, but the shoreline regression rate and the distance of seaward sediment transport (Figure 9b) are different. This could be caused by the different natures of low-frequency waves. Waves of low-frequency bands can include infragravity waves (IGW) of different kinds: bound long waves and break point-forced long waves [6]. Previous investigations have shown show that various IGW affect the coast in two different ways: a) bound long waves protect the shore, b) the break-point forces long waves, leading to an intensification of near-shore erosion [28].

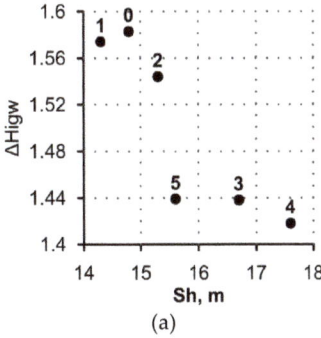 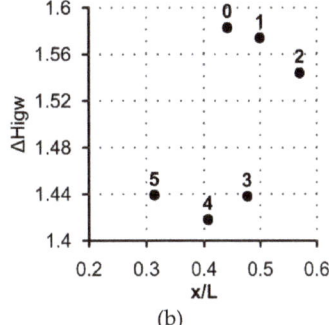

Figure 9. Dependence of (**a**) the shoreline retreat (Sh, m) and (**b**) the relative distance of seaward sediment transport (x/L)over a on relative change in mean wave period (ΔTmean, s) occurring during wave transformation over a barred profile (620–820 m, see Figure 4). L is the wavelength calculated for deep-water conditions, x is the distance of the maximal sediments transported away from the shore.

The presence of the underwater bar changed the symmetry of the waves. The wave skewness, after passing the bar (the x-coordinate on the profile was 820 m), remained almost similar ≈ 1.6 for all profiles. High values of the skewness coefficient show that breaking in XBeach model is probably described as spilling, because in observations and laboratory experiments plunging breaking waves have skewness less than 1 [29]. Waves breaking by spillage are symmetric relative to the vertical axis, they have sharp crests and flat troughs, while plunging breaking waves have steep fronts [30].

The wave asymmetry coefficient behaves differently. Figure 10 shows the wave asymmetry coefficient in a nearshore area (the 820 m coordinate on the profile) and its relation with shoreline regression and seaward sediment transport distance. According to the model data, the more asymmetric waves are after the bar, the less the coastline degrades.

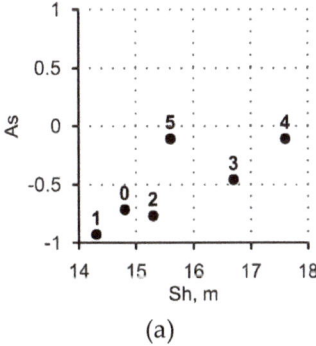 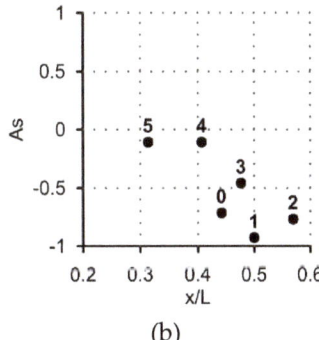

Figure 10. Dependence of (**a**) shoreline retreat (Sh, m) and (**b**) the relative distance of seaward sediment transport (x/L) on wave asymmetry (As) after wave transformation (near the shore, at the x-coordinate 820 m). L is the wavelength calculated for deep-water conditions, and x is the distance of maximal sediments transported away from the shore.

The most asymmetric waves behind the bar were observed on profiles where the first wave breaking occurred, between the coast and the bar, for example, on profiles with the bar's distant location (profiles 1 and 2), as well as on a profile without a bar (profile 0, see Figure 3). When the bar was located closer to the shore, and accordingly, the depth decreased above it, the waves broke both at the top of the bar, and near the shore. In this case, the waves broke over the bar farther from the shore than on the profiles 0–2, and the second breaking zone was closer to the coastline. The presence of two breaking points leads to a significantly greater shoreline regression. The exception for this is the profile 5, where the bar is located at the closest distance to the coast line. The bar prevents seaward sediment transport, so that the shoreline degradation is reduced.

An Explanation of wave asymmetry impact on sediment transport w discussed in detail in [30]. Cross-shore sediment transport is defined by the balance of wav- induced sediment transport directed to the shore, and the undertow, which moves sediments seaward. According to Bailard's formulation of wave-induced sediment transport discharge [31] depends on highest statistical moments of near bottom velocity:

$$q = \frac{1}{2} f_w \rho \left(\frac{\varepsilon_b}{\tan \Phi} \overline{u|u|^2} + \frac{\varepsilon_s}{W_s} \overline{u|u|^3} \right) \qquad (7)$$

where u = u(t): the instantaneous near-bottom velocity.

Formula (7) was adopted by Leontiev [6] for calculations through amplitudes of first and second nonlinear harmonics of near bottom-velocity and cosines of phase lag between them (bi-phases):

$$\overline{u|u|^2} = \frac{3}{4} u_m^2 u_{2m} \cos \beta, \quad \overline{u|u|^3} = \frac{16}{5\pi} u_m^3 u_{2m} \cos \beta \qquad (8)$$

where u_m and u_{2m} – amplitudes of first and second harmonics, β- phase shift between the first and second nonlinear harmonics (bi-phases).

As it was revealed in [31], the wave asymmetry coefficient As was linear, depends on bi-phase:

$$As = 0.8\beta \qquad (9)$$

Thus, according to (8 and 9), the shoreward wave induced-sediment discharge depends on the cosine of the bi-phase, or As magnitude. Maximum of it will occur when bi-phase (and accordingly As) is zero, because cosine will has maximal value. A decrease of wave-induced sediment discharge due to wave asymmetry will lead to increase in the role of the undertow in sediment transport. Therefore, sediments will move more seaward, and the shoreline will retreat more, due to the erosion in nearshore zones (see Figure 10b).

4. Conclusions

We carried out a study on the influence of the underwater bar location on the transformation of the waves above it, and on the corresponding cross-shore sediment movement in the coastal zone, on a time scale of one storm. This allows us to conclude on the following:

1. The position of the underwater bar affects the shoreline degradation and the distance of seaward sediment transport. The maximum transfer of sediments towards the sea is within the distance between the shoreline and the underwater bar crest. A minimum of sediment movement occurs when the bar is located away from the shore, at a distance of less than half the wavelength, in deep water. The coastline retreat is minimal if the bar is located away from the coast, at a distance of 0.7-0.82 from the wavelength in deep water. In these cases, the underwater bar will have a more protective effect on the shore, compared to a profile without the bar.

2. The presence of the underwater bar located at specific distances from the coast may lead to an increase in shoreline degradation. If there is a longshore underwater bar that is located at an angle to the coastline, the non-uniformity of the coastline retreat, and the formation of festoons are possible.

3. The greatest difference in coastal retreat rate associated with the underwater bar location is observed within the first hour of the storm. Regardless of the location of the underwater bar on the initial profile, the equilibrium profile is formed after 6 h, for the selected wave conditions. The resulting equilibrium profile contains an underwater terrace, and it is close to the classical equilibrium profile. At the same time, the erosion rate slows down significantly and becomes identical for all profiles.

4. Changing the parameters of the waves during their transformation over different profiles has a significant impact on the degree of transformation of the underwater beach profile. It has

been established that there is an inverse relationship between the retreat of the coast line and the low-frequency wave heights near the coast. The decrease in the mean wave period, which is associated with the growth of higher harmonics during the passage of waves above the bar, reduces shoreline erosion. The distance of seaward sediment transport transfer is directly related to the significant wave height.

5. When waves propagate over profiles with underwater bars that are located at different distances from the coast, the wave asymmetry changes differently. According to the modelling results, the increase in wave asymmetry near the shore due to the existence of the bar leads to a decrease in the influence of waves on the coastal retreat.

Author Contributions: Both authors took part in field works on Shkorpilovtsy study site. XBeach modelling was conducted by O.K. in frame of post-graduate study (Y.S. was a scientific advisor). Analysis of modelling data was carried out by O.K. and Y.S.

Funding: This research was performed in the framework of the state assignment theme No. 0149-2019-0005, and supported in part by RFBR project No. 18-55-45026.

Acknowledgments: Authors appreciate collaboration with colleagues from IO BAS (Varna, Bulgaria) and Zenkovich laboratory of the sea shelf and coasts (IO RAS, Moscow, Russia).

Conflicts of Interest: The authors declare no conflict of interest.

References

1. Cheng, J.; Wang, P.; Smith, E.R. Hydrodynamic conditions associated with an onshore migrating and stable sandbar. *J. Coast. Res.* **2016**, *32*, 153–163.
2. Salem, A.S.; Jarno-Druaux, A.; Marin, F. Physical modeling of cross-shore beach morphodynamics under waves and tides. *J. Coast. Res.* **2011**, *SI 64*, 139–143.
3. Grasso, F.; Michallet, H.; Certain, R.; Barthélemy, E. Experimental Flume Simulation of Sandbar Dynamics. *J. Coast. Res.* **2009**, *1*, 54–58.
4. Leont'ev, O.K. *Morskaja Geologija (Osnovy Geologii i Geomorfologii Mirovogo Okeana). Marine Geology (Fundamentals of Geology and Geomorphology of the World Ocean)*; Vysshee Obrazovanie: Moscow, Russia, 1982. (In Russian)
5. Ruessink, B.G.; Wijnberg, K.M.; Holman, R.A.; Kuriyama, Y.; van Enckevort, I.M.J. Intersite comparison of interannual nearshore bar behaviour. *J. Geophys. Res.* **2003**, *108*. [CrossRef]
6. Leont'ev, I.O. *Pribrezhnaja Dinamika: Volny, Techenija, Potoki Nanosov (Coastal Dynamics: Waves, Currents, Sediment Flows)*; GEOS: Moskva, Russia, 2001. (In Russian)
7. Briganti, R.; Musumeci, R.E.; van der Meer, J.; Romano, A.; Stancanelli, L.M.; Kudella, M.; Akbar, R.; Mukhdiar, R.; Altomare, C.; Suzuki, T.; et al. Large scale tests on foreshore evolution during storm sequences and the performance of a nearly vertical structure. *Coast. Eng. Proc.* **2018**, *1*, 13. [CrossRef]
8. *Proektirovanie Morskih Beregozashchitnyh Sooruzhenij (Design of Offshore Protective Structures)*; SP 32-103-97; Korporaciya «TRANSSTROJ»: Moscow, Russia, 1998. (In Russian)
9. Saprykina, Y.; Kuznetsov, S.; Korzinin, D. Nonlinear transformation of waves above submerged structures. *Procedia Eng.* **2015**, *116*, 187–194. [CrossRef]
10. Abanades, J.; Greaves, D.; Iglesias, G. Coastal defence through wave farms. *Coast. Eng.* **2014**, *91*, 299–307. [CrossRef]
11. Kuznetsova, O.; Saprykina, Y.; Shtremel, M.; Kuznetsov, S.; Korzinin, D.; Trifonova, E.; Andreeva, N.; Valchev, N.; Prodanov, B.; Eftimova, P. Dynamics of sandy beach in dependence on wave parameters. In Proceedings of the IMAM2017 Conference: Maritime Transportation and Harvesting of Sea Resources, Lisbon, Portugal, 9–10 October 2017; Tailor and Francis Group: London, UK, 2017; pp. 1075–1079, ISBN 978-0-8153-7993-5.
12. *Dynamical Processes in Coastal Regions. Results of the Kamchiya International Project*; IO BAS: Sofia, Bulgaria, 1990.
13. XBeach Open Source Community. Available online: https://oss.deltares.nl/web/xbeach (accessed on 5 February 2019).

14. Hartanto, I.M.; Beevers, L.; Popescu, I.; Wright, N.G. Application of a coastal modelling code in fluvial environments. *Environ. Model. Softw.* **2011**, *26*, 1685–1695. [CrossRef]
15. Saponieri, A.; Di Risio, M.; Pasquali, D.; Valentini, N.; Aristodemo, F.; Tripepi, G.; Celli, D.; Streicher, M.; Damiani, L. Beach profile evolution in front of storm seawalls: A physical and numerical study. *Coast. Eng. Proc.* **2018**, *1*, 70. [CrossRef]
16. Roelvink, D.; Reniers, A.; van Dongeren, A.; van Thiel de Vries, J.; McCall, R.; Lescinski, J. Modelling storm impacts on beaches, dunes and barrier islands. *Coast. Eng.* **2009**, *56*, 1133–1152. [CrossRef]
17. Kuznetsova, O.A.; Saprykina, J.V.; Trifonova, E.V. Jeksperimental'nye issledovanija vlijanija volnenija na deformacii rel'efa dna beregovoj zony (Experimental research of wave impact on coastal relief deformation). *Processy v Geosredah* **2015**, *2*, 66–74. (In Russian)
18. *Spravochnye Dannye po Rezhimu vetra i Volnenija Baltijskogo, Severnogo, Chernogo, Azovskogo i Sredizemnogo Morej (Information on Wind-Wave Regime of Baltic, North, Black, Asov and Mediterranean Seas*; Rossijskij Morskoj Registr Sudohodstva: St. Petersburg, Russia, 2006. (In Russian)
19. Valchev, N.N.; Trifonova, E.V.; Andreeva, N.K. Past and recent trends in the western Black Sea storminess. *Nat. Hazards Earth Syst. Sci.* **2012**, *12*, 961–977. [CrossRef]
20. Roelvink, D.; McCall, R.; Mehvar, S.; Nederhoff, K.; Dastgheib, A. Improving predictions of swash dynamics in XBeach: The role of groupiness and incident-band runup. *Coast. Eng.* **2018**, *134*, 103–123. [CrossRef]
21. Elsayed, S.M.; Oumeraci, H. Effect of beach slope and grain-stabilization on coastal sediment transport: An attempt to overcome the erosion overestimation by XBeach. *Coast. Eng.* **2017**, *121*, 179–196. [CrossRef]
22. Naumova, V.A.; Evstigneev, M.P.; Evstigneev, V.P.; Lybarets, E.P. Vetro-volnovye uslovija Azovo-Chernomorskogo poberezh'ja Ukrainy (Wind-wave conditions of Azov and Black Sea coast of Ukraine). *Nauk. Praci UkrNDGMI* **2010**, *259*, 263–283. (In Russian)
23. Belberov, Z.; Davidan, I.; Kostichkova, D.; Lavrenov, I.; Lopatukhin, L.; Cherneva, Z. Main principles for creation of a new wind-wave atlas of the Bulgarian sector of the Black Sea. *Proc. IO-BAS Varna* **1992**, *1*, 5–12. (In Bulgarian)
24. Lozano, I.; Devoy, R.J.N.; May, W.; Andersen, U. Storminess and vulnerability along the Atlantic coastlines of Europe: Analysis of storm records and of a greenhouse gases induced climate scenario. *Mar. Geol.* **2004**, *210*, 205–225. [CrossRef]
25. *Guide to Wave Analysis and Forecasting*; WMO-No.702; WMO: Geneva, Switzerland, 1992; 159p.
26. *Coastal Engineering Manual*; Engineer Manual 1110-2-1100; U.S. Army Corps of Engineers: Washington, DC, USA, 2002; Volume 6.
27. Dean, R.G. Equilibrium beach profiles: Characteristics and applications. *J. Coast. Res.* **1990**, *7*, 53–84.
28. Kuznetsova, O.; Saprykina, Y.; Divinsky, B. Underwater barred beach profile transformation under different waves conditions. In Proceedings of the International Conference "Managing Risks to Coastal Regions and Communities in a Changing World" (EMECS'11—SeaCoasts XXVI), St. Petersburg, Russia, 22–27 August 2016; RIOR Publ.: Moscow, Russia, 2016.
29. Saprykina, Y.V.; Kuznetsov, S.Y.; Divinskii, B.V. Influence of processes of nonlinear transformations of waves in the coastal zone on the height of breaking waves. *Oceanology* **2017**, *57*, 383–393. [CrossRef]
30. Kuznetsov, S.; Saprykina, Y.; Shtremel, M.; Kuznetsova, O. Spectral structure of breaking waves and its possible influence on the transport of sediments in coastal zone. In Proceedings of the Conference "Oceans'15 MTS/IEEE Genova", Genova, Italy, 18–21 May 2015.
31. Bailard, J.A. An energetic total load sediment transport model for a plane sloping beach. *J. Geophys. Res. Oceans* **1981**, *86*, 10938–10954. [CrossRef]

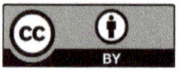

© 2019 by the authors. Licensee MDPI, Basel, Switzerland. This article is an open access article distributed under the terms and conditions of the Creative Commons Attribution (CC BY) license (http://creativecommons.org/licenses/by/4.0/).

MDPI
St. Alban-Anlage 66
4052 Basel
Switzerland
Tel. +41 61 683 77 34
Fax +41 61 302 89 18
www.mdpi.com

Journal of Marine Science and Engineering Editorial Office
E-mail: jmse@mdpi.com
www.mdpi.com/journal/jmse

www.ingramcontent.com/pod-product-compliance
Lightning Source LLC
LaVergne TN
LVHW070551100526
838202LV00012B/435